GET PREPPED STAGE READY FITNESS

FIRST EDITION

ISBN: 9781916247178

Printed in the United States

Library of Congress Cataloging-in-Publication Data

© 2019 All rights reserved

This program is fully copyrighted and does not come with giveaway or resale rights.

You may not sell or redistribute this program. Copyright and illegal distribution violations will be prosecuted.

CONTENTS

DISCLAIMER

This program is designed for healthy individuals over 18 years old, and the information should be used in conjunction with the guidance and care of your physician or an equally qualified Health Care Professional.

By taking part in this program and using any of the recommendations within it, you are agreeing to behave responsibility and accept full responsibility for your actions.

By continuing with the program you recognise that despite all precautions on the part of DreamGirl Fitness™, there are risks of injury or illness which can occur because of your use of the aforementioned information and you expressly assume such risks and waive, remise, discharge, relinquish and release any claim which you may have against DreamGirl Fitness™, or its affiliates, joint ventures, partners, contractors, or independent contractors as a result of any future physical injury or illness incurred in connection with, or as a result of, the use or misuse of the program.

This is a complete and conditional release of all liability to the greatest extent allowed by law and agree that if any portion of this Terms, Conditions, Waiver and Releases is held to be invalid, the balance, notwithstanding, shall continue in full force and effect.

If your physician recommends you not to use the DreamCurves™ program, please listen to your physician and follow this advice.

SUCCESS TRACKING

Before you start the program, you will need to take:

+ Starting weight
+ Body fat pinch
+ Measurements
+ Photos

During the first 4 weeks, you will be checking your progress weekly. This will ensure that you are on the right nutrition amount for you. Following this initial period, you may drop back to once every other week or every three weeks according to your preference.

To keep you accountable, you will be checking your progress the day after your refeed meal. This will ensure you don't go overboard.

Set yourself a reminder on your phone each week so you don't forget to check in. This is your accountability and motivation throughout the journey, and you'll be much more likely to stick to the program if you maintain an active interest in logging your progress.

SCALE WEIGHT

Ugh, scales. Those dreaded horrible things that think it's fun to mess with your mind every day.

The reason why scales are so bad is because they don't tell the whole story and they do lie. It's comparable to reading one line of text and then taking the whole book out of context based on that one piece of information.

Your body is made up of more than just fat, so why is one number on the scale soul destroying for so many people? Let's say you burnt off your liver while you were out running and then went to weigh yourself to find you're 6lb lighter. Surely that wouldn't make you jump for joy, or at least I hope not. But this is what's happening every day. Okay, the liver was a bit over the top, but it's not all that far off either. People are jumping for joy because of the number reflected on this contraption, never mind that they may have lost precious muscle.

Conversely, let's say you've been training hard for a few weeks and you've lost 4lbs of fat, but you've gained 5lbs of muscle. On the scale, you've gained a pound and it looks like a failed few weeks, however, in reality your body is looking tighter and more toned because your composition has changed.

IT'S ABOUT COMPOSITION

The sad thing is, I have known guys and girls who have taken laxatives or made themselves purge just so they could reduce the number on the scale. It's not right.

Where the weight is coming from is so important if you want to sport a hard and toned sexy body and not a thin, bony starved looking one because if that weight is coming from your precious lean tissue, the stuff that keeps your body strong and healthy, it's more than likely your fat is actually sticking around.

Sure you can purchase fancy body composition scales now, but they're worse. The readings are all over the place. When I was at my leanest before my show, the composition scales I used threw back 25%. It's just plain wrong and could be making a lot of people sick.

Still not convinced? Check out the guidance on Skinny fat syndrome to learn more about body composition and it's effect on how your book looks. I'm sure you'll be convinced soon after.

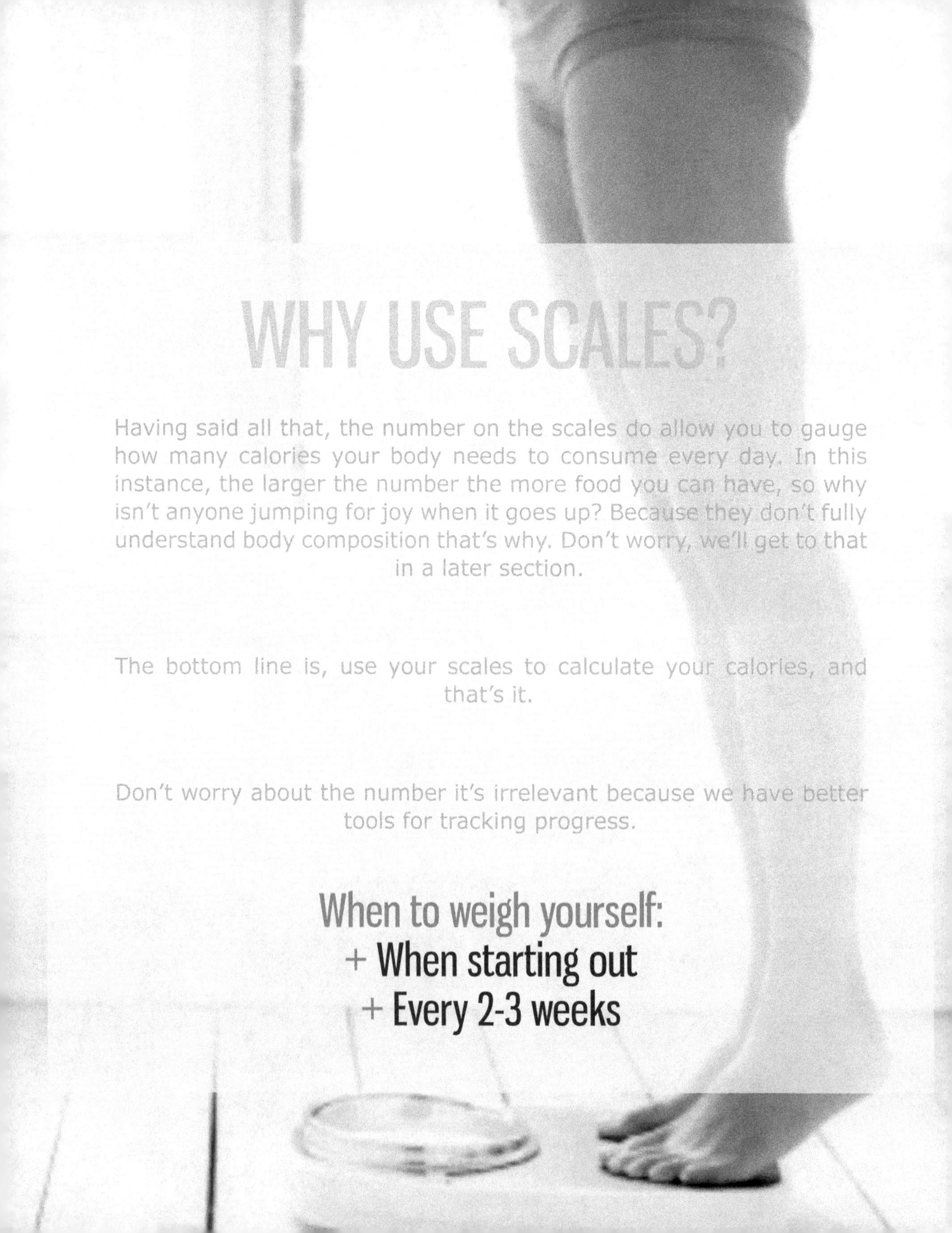

WHY USE SCALES?

Having said all that, the number on the scales do allow you to gauge how many calories your body needs to consume every day. In this instance, the larger the number the more food you can have, so why isn't anyone jumping for joy when it goes up? Because they don't fully understand body composition that's why. Don't worry, we'll get to that in a later section.

The bottom line is, use your scales to calculate your calories, and that's it.

Don't worry about the number it's irrelevant because we have better tools for tracking progress.

When to weigh yourself:

+ When starting out
+ Every 2-3 weeks

BODY FAT CALLIPERS

The next most popular way of tracking progress is with body fat callipers. Callipers sort of resemble a medieval torture device, but they are painless. You simply pinch your flesh and measure the thickness. The reading displayed is the one you want to record. Simple.

When you purchase the calipers, they'll come with detailed instructions on their usage, so I'll not delve into thos here. Just be sure to follow the instructions for accuracy.

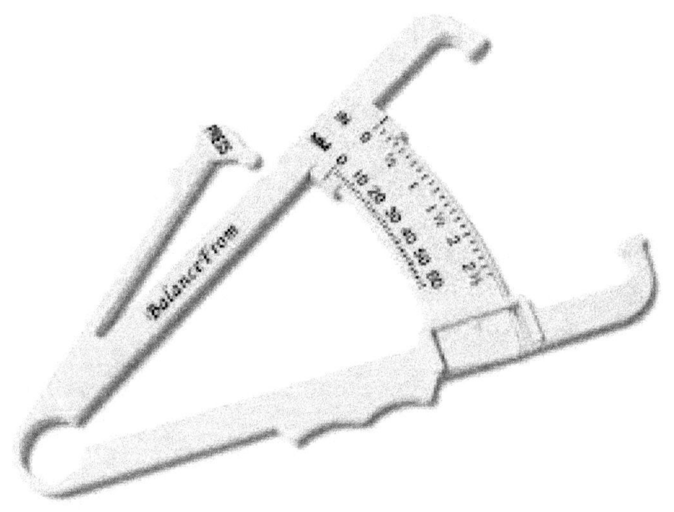

KEEP IT CONSISTENT

These are a great tool and are far better than scales, however, these can also have their share of problems. The reliability of the results depend on the skills of the person taking the reading, as well as consistency in the location the readings are taken from. Therefore, when using the callipers, it is important to take the reading as consistently as possible. Pinch the same location on your body and take 3 readings to get an average.

Just like the scales, callipers don't tell the whole story because flesh is made up of both fat and water, however, this is still a great and inexpensive tool to use, and one I highly recommend getting to grips with.

RECOMMENDED CALLIPER

+ Accu Measure Personal Body Fat Tester

Instructions come with the calliper, follow those as closely as possible.

WHEN TO MEASURE YOURSELF

+ When starting out

+ Every 2-3 weeks

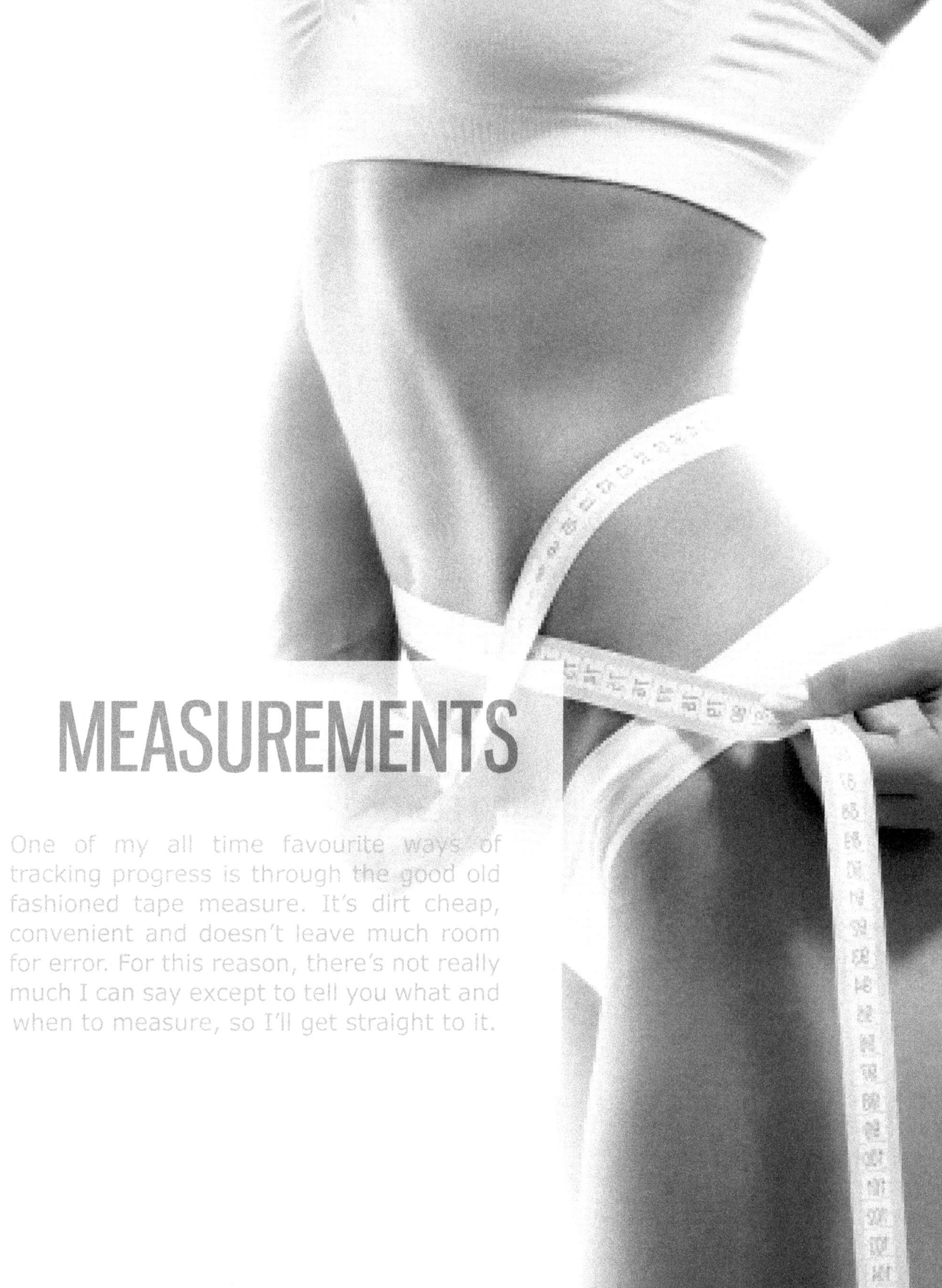

MEASUREMENTS

One of my all time favourite ways of tracking progress is through the good old fashioned tape measure. It's dirt cheap, convenient and doesn't leave much room for error. For this reason, there's not really much I can say except to tell you what and when to measure, so I'll get straight to it.

TAKING THE MEASUREMENTS

POINTS TO NOTE

Be sure to remain consistent in your measuring, always measure as closely as possible to the previous point.

Measure snugly, but not so tight that it compresses the skin as this will distort the measurement.

WHEN TO MEASURE YOURSELF

+ When starting out
+ Every 2-3 weeks

WHAT TO MEASURE

Shoulders

Measure the widest part, shoulder to shoulder

Chest

Measure just above the nipple

Bicep

Measure the left or right, but be consistent each time. Measure un-flexed

Waist

Measure at the belly button. Do not suck your stomach in

Hips

Measure the widest point

Thigh

Measure the left or right, but be consistent each time

Calf

Measure the widest point

PHOTOGRAPHS

Photos are by far the greatest progress tool ever. Not only do they give you feedback, they are also visual so you can see with your own eyes what you may not be seeing in mirror every day. Photos are motivating, and they are pretty accurate provided they are done with consistency.

In the beginning, you may feel a bit uncomfortable. That's fine and perfectly natural. You can even look at them in disgust and use that as your motivation, or you can take them, don't look and hide them in a folder on your computer until you have progressed into the program for a few weeks. It's up to you, but please take them as you'll regret it if you don't, trust me.

TIPS FOR SUCCESS

WEAR SOMETHING SMALL

You need to see skin, it's that simple. When your body changes, body parts begin to lift, cellulite diminish, and skin tightens. How will you see any of these things if you are camouflaged behind clothing? You can't, so find a bathing suit and use that as your progress suit.

CLEAR ENVIRONMENT

Try to keep clutter out of the photo with a solid backdrop, and keep the light as evenly distributed as possible to avoid hard shadows. Natural light is best.

HANDS FREE IF POSSIBLE

Hands free if possible:

This may not be possible, but if you can take photos hands free, you'll be able to remain consistent with your photos so much easier. You can ask a friend or relative, or use a tripod with a timer. You could also use a video camera function which is actually a pretty great way of seeing progress too, and you can take screenshots when you play it back. Mirror selfies are difficult to track, I've made that mistake myself.

USE STANDARD POSES

+ Front Stand relaxed, hands by your side

+Back Stand relaxed, hands by your side

+Sides Stand relaxed, arms raised in front. Take both sides

BE CONSISTENT

Take the photo under the same conditions each time. So, if you take them first thing in the morning in your bathing suit, you always take them first thing in the morning in that same bathing suit. You can take photos all day long of your body parts, but these are your official progress photos that you'll use to track progress, so keep them consistent, no special poses, no fancy lighting setups, jus the same conditions all the time. Okay, I think you get my point.

WHEN TO TAKE PHOTOS

+ When starting out
+ Every 1-2 weeks

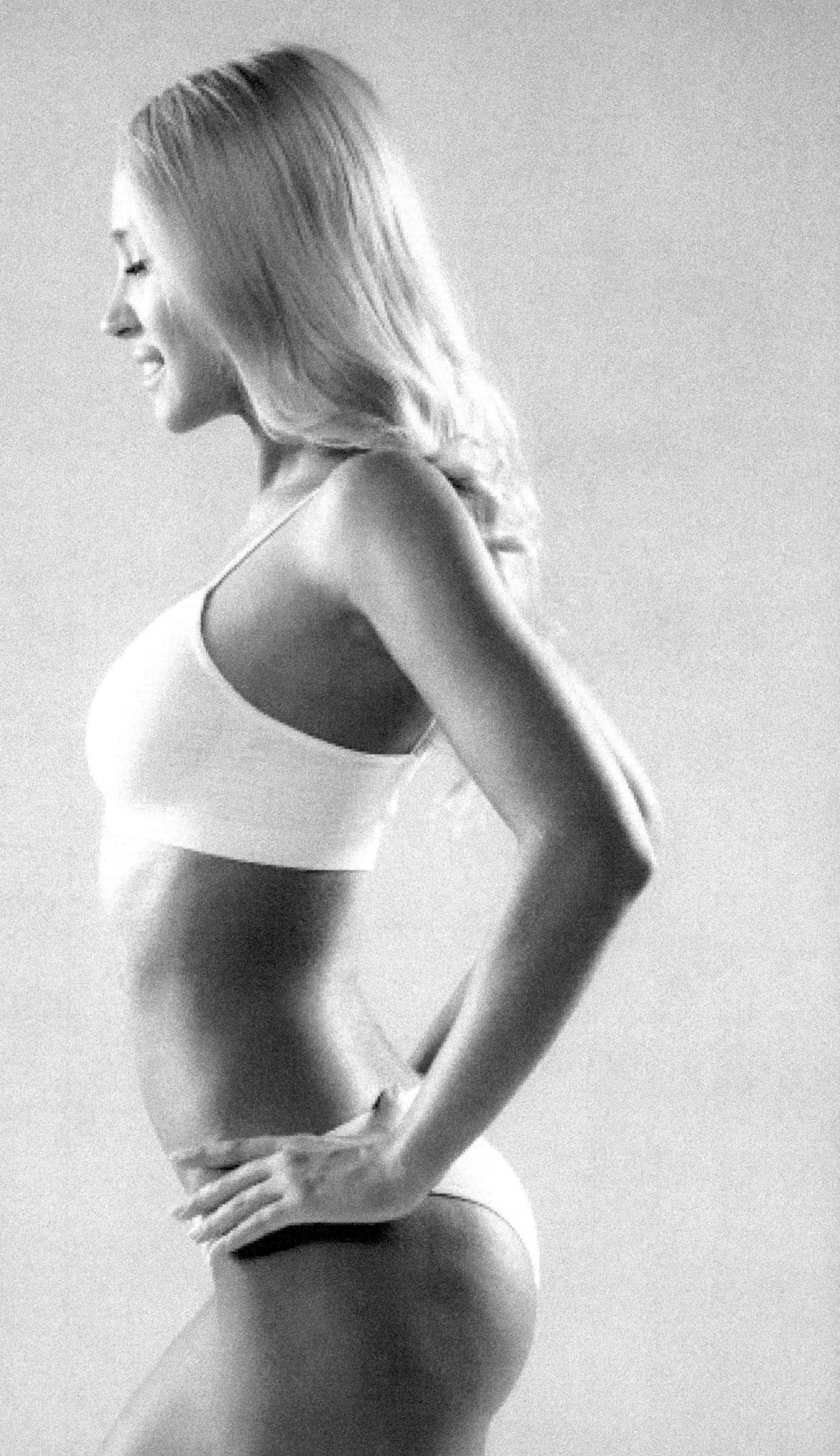

VISUAL COMPARISON

Here is a visual guide that can also help you assess and compare your progress. Rather than going by numbers alone.

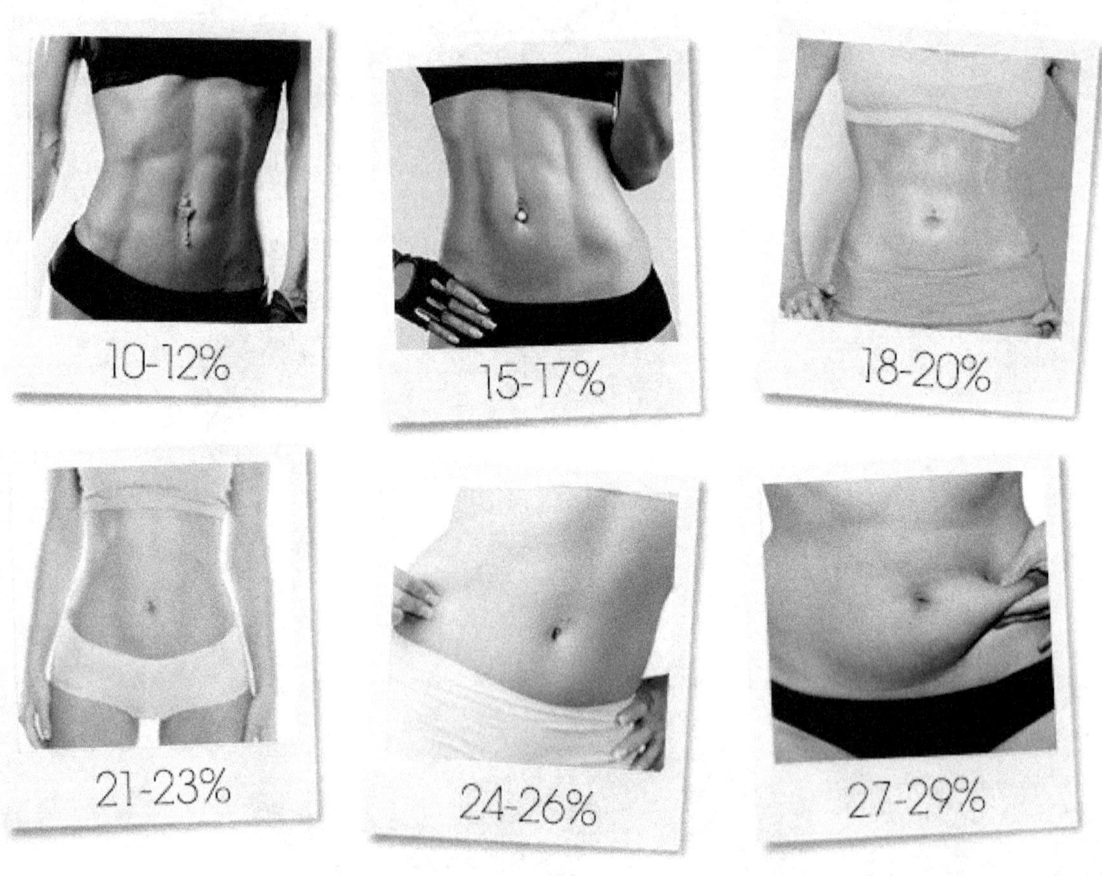

TRACK YOUR TRAINING

If you fail to track your lifting, you'll never progress. I know this because this is exactly where I started.

When I finally realised that 5-10 miles of cardio a day wasn't the key to my DreamGirl curves, my boyfriend offered to teach me some basic lifts. Unfortunately, he didn't tell me about keeping track and increasing the weights each week, and I didn't know to ask. I started lifting and all was good, for a while. My arms started looking shapelier by the week, my shoulders developed that cute little dimple at the top, and I was super happy to see myself making progress.

Each week I picked up around about the same weights and performed as much as I could be bothered to do. I'm not even sure what rep range I was using. Let's just say that it wasn't very well thought out. Boy was I naive and uneducated back then. Sigh...

WHY IT'S SO IMPORTANT

After a few months of lifting, I started to notice that those initial improvements had stopped. Each week I took a progress photo, I was disappointed to find the same body reflected back at me. So, in my frustration and without any knowledge of what I was doing, I did what anyone would do: I reduced my calories and carbs and started taking so called miracle thermogenic compounds. Oh dear. Gasp. Need I say, it didn't work and I ended up giving up, for a while.

I have since smartened up a whole lot and have learned that tracking progress is not only nice for your sense of accomplishment and bragging rights, it is also essential if you actually want to see some changes taking place. Now, unless you've signed up to this program for a bit of fun, which I doubt, you want solid and measurable progress. In which case, you're going to have to track your training It's really that simple.

If you are tracking your numbers, you'll always know if you're heading in the right direction. No numbers and you may as well flip a coin and hope for the best. The good news is I've created some convenient printable journal pages for you to track it all in.

WHAT TO TRACK

Within your journal pages, you'll be able to track the following training aspects:

+ Exercise performed
+ Reps performed per set
+ Weight used
+ Supporting notes

Supporting notes can be very useful for keeping track of things such your rest, mood, diet, energy levels, time of the month, etc. As you continue on your training program, you'll be thankful for such notes as you may begin to see patterns in your progress which can can help you bust out of a plateau.

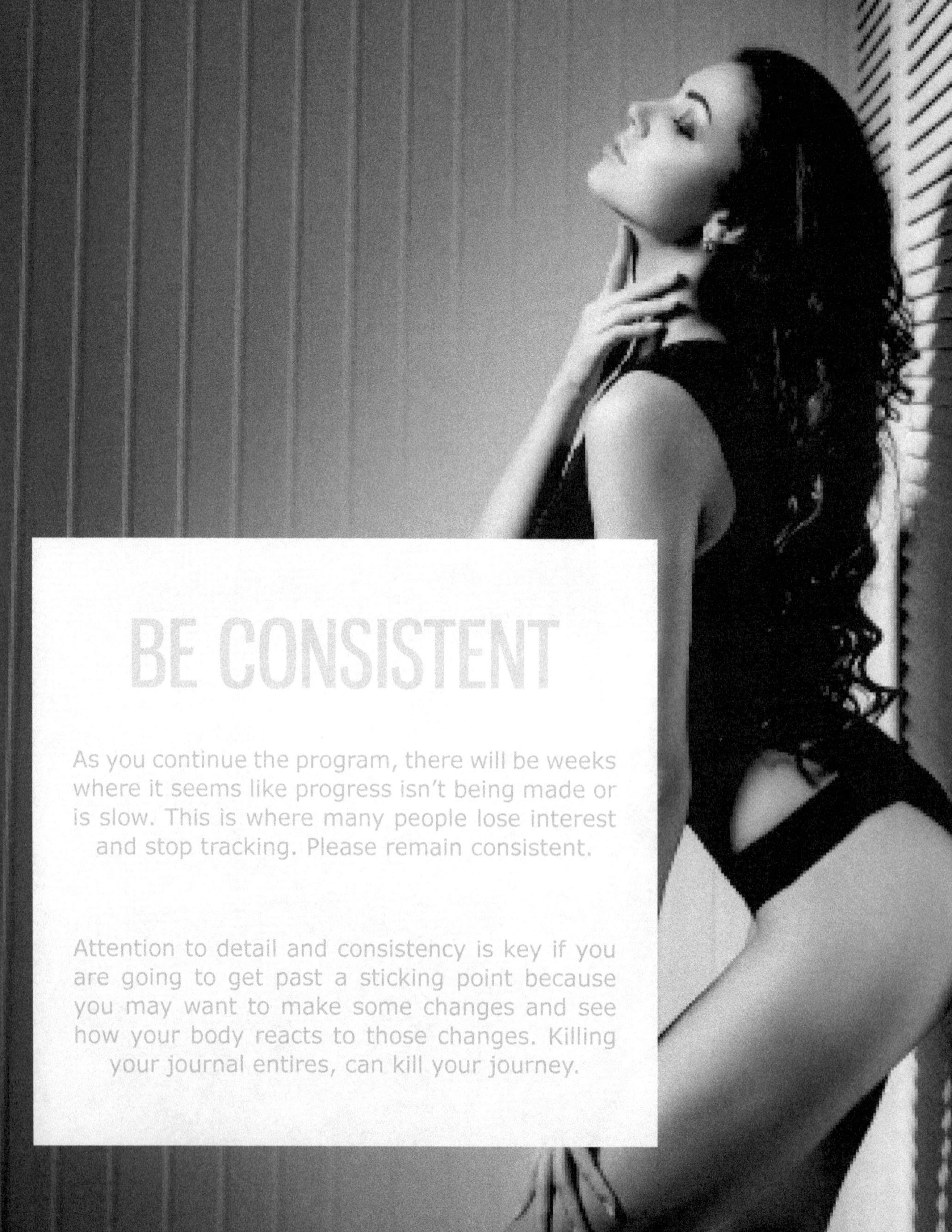

BE CONSISTENT

As you continue the program, there will be weeks where it seems like progress isn't being made or is slow. This is where many people lose interest and stop tracking. Please remain consistent.

Attention to detail and consistency is key if you are going to get past a sticking point because you may want to make some changes and see how your body reacts to those changes. Killing your journal entires, can kill your journey.

IT'S ALL ABOUT YOU

This system wouldn't be complete without first understanding you and your individual needs, so that's where we begin the program. First we will take a look at your body shape and type, and then we determine the best approach for you.

While it isn't possible to change your genetics, it is possible through the correct execution of exercise and a balanced approach to sculpt and manipulate your body to give the illusion of a shapely hourglass shape, and that is the purpose of this program. Through our unique approach and understanding of your body characteristics, the DreamCurves™ program utilises carefully selected and targeted training techniques to create a program that works for you, and therefore get you the results your aspire to.

So, let's take a look at the different body shapes.

MESOMORPH

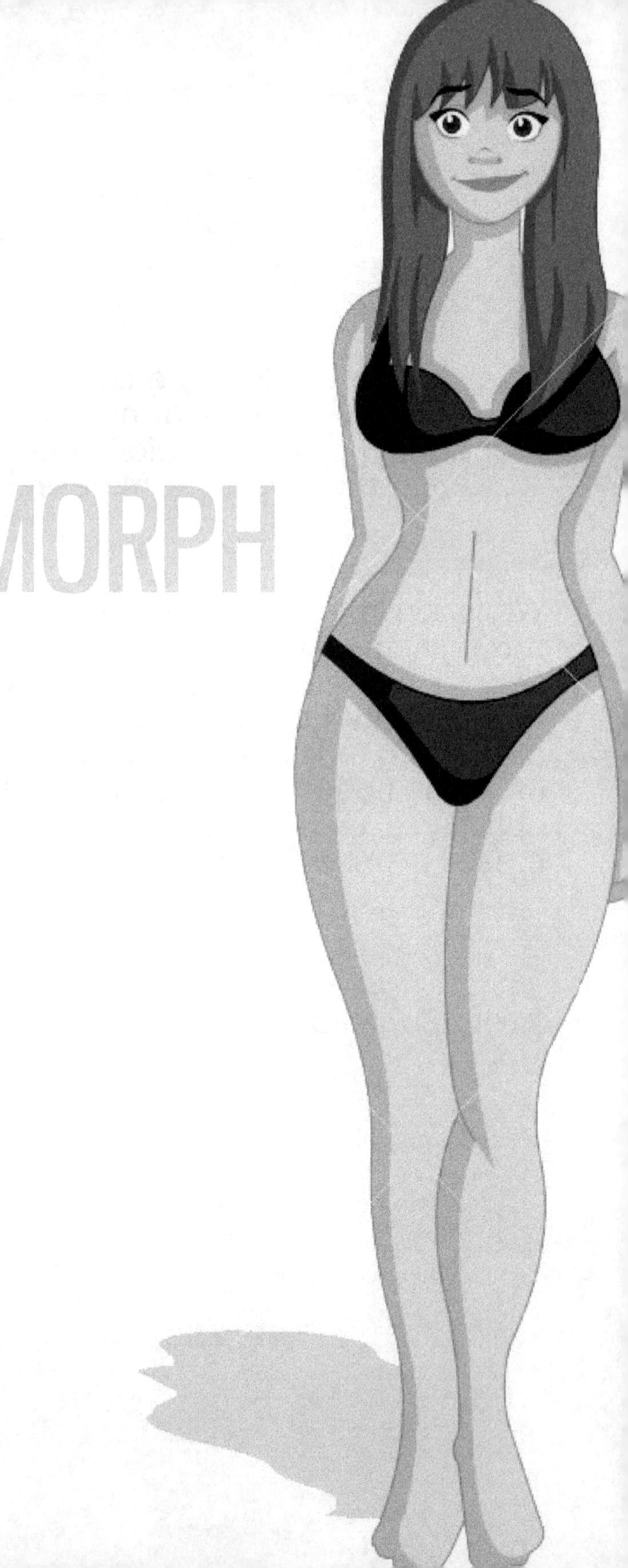

Mesomorphs are often described as genetically gifted. They have efficient metabolisms, so don't have to worry too much about what they eat, and they tend to be relatively muscular without much effort, which gives them an athletic and strong appearance, and excellent definition.

They tend to be well proportioned all over, tending to store fat evenly throughout their bodies. They are often characterised by strong bones, thick thighs, and appear blessed with curves.

+ Medium size joints and bones
+ Naturally lean and lose fat easily
+ Naturally muscular and gain muscle readily
+ Naturally strong and responds quickly to exercise
+ Have plenty of curves and shape

As this body type gains muscle relatively easily, care should be taken to introduce the correct targeted weight training, so not to increase muscular size and bulk in the wrong areas. The good news is that sculpting out a super sexy feminine shape will be easiest for you. The bad news is, sculpting the wrong shape can be just as easy with the wrong approach. Lucky you are a DreamGirl.

ECTOMORPH

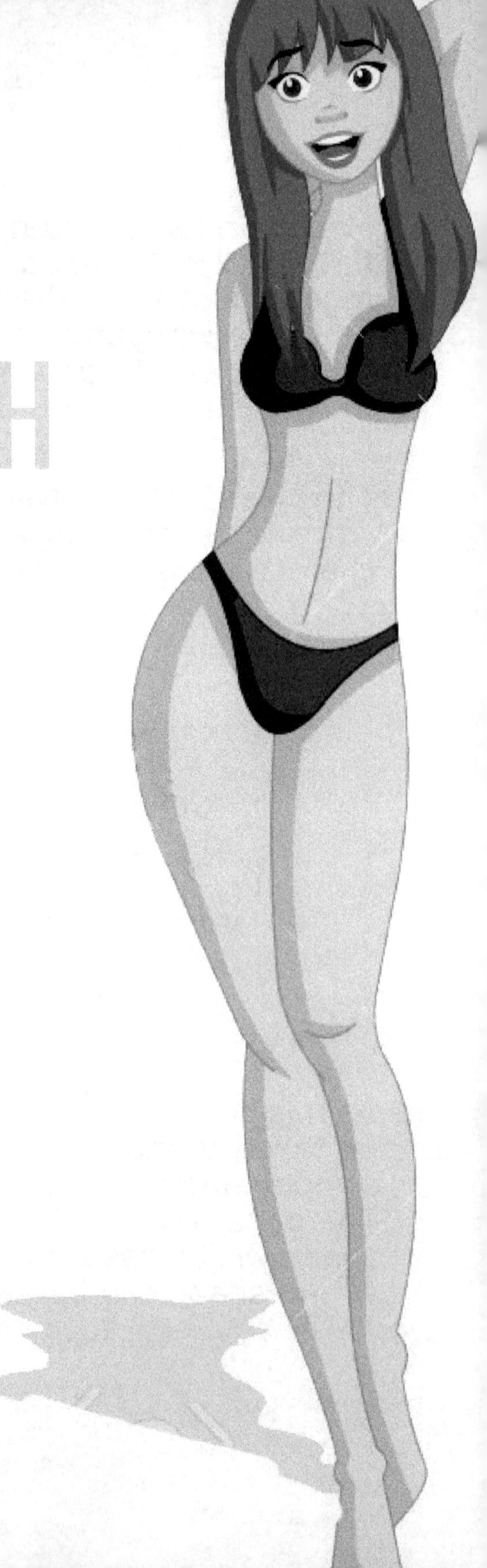

Ectomorphs have fast and efficient metabolisms, and therefore tend to be naturally slim and wiry. They have difficulties in gaining weight and adding lean muscle mass, even without exercising and dieting. Ectomorphs are often flat chested, lack curves and are slightly boyish in shape.

Models, ballerina's and basketball players are characteristic of ectomorph qualities, which can be defined as:

+ Slim joints and bones
+ Fragile and delicate bodies
+ Long limbs
+ Linear body shape
+ Small shoulders
+ Small chest and buttocks
+ Little muscle mass

The focus of this body type is on gaining lean muscle mass through a mass building diet and heavy weight training. The good news is body fat will remain naturally low, so any new definition will be immediately visible and there will be little need for cardio to keep body fat levels low. The bad news, you'll have to work hard to get those curves.

ENDOMORPH

Endomorphs have a sluggish metabolism so gain weight easily and, therefore, tend to appear soft and curvy. That being said, endomorphs also gain muscle easily, so an in shape endomorph appears very feminine and sexy with plenty of curves.

+ Medium to large joints and frame
+ Smooth and round body
+ Short limbs
+ High levels of body fat
+ Gains muscle easily
+ Loses weight slowly

Because an endomorphs metabolism is unforgiving, focus is primarily on lowering body fat levels. This can be achieved through HIIT training and a lower intake of carbohydrates. The good news is that sculpting a beautiful and sexy hourglass shape will be easy for you. The bad news, you'll have to work hard to show off those curves.

IDENTIFY

While weight distribution plays a vital role in how your body shape appears, your basic underlying structure may be different. If your excess body fat goes straight to your hips and thighs for instance, you may appear to be pear shaped, where in fact you may be hourglass beneath it all. This is why a lean body is essential to this program.

To determine your shape, strip down to your underwear and look at yourself straight on in the mirror. Place your hands and arms a little away from your sides, and legs together. Examine the area under your arms, your bust and ribcage, your waist and hips, and determine the fullest part. Take a look at the following characteristics to determine the closest match.

It is possible to fall between the shapes, so a bit of judgement from you will be needed.

PEAR SHAPE

The pear, aka triangle, shape is characteris

+ Full hips and thighs
+ Narrow shoulders
+ Smaller bust
+ Wear a larger size on bottom vs your

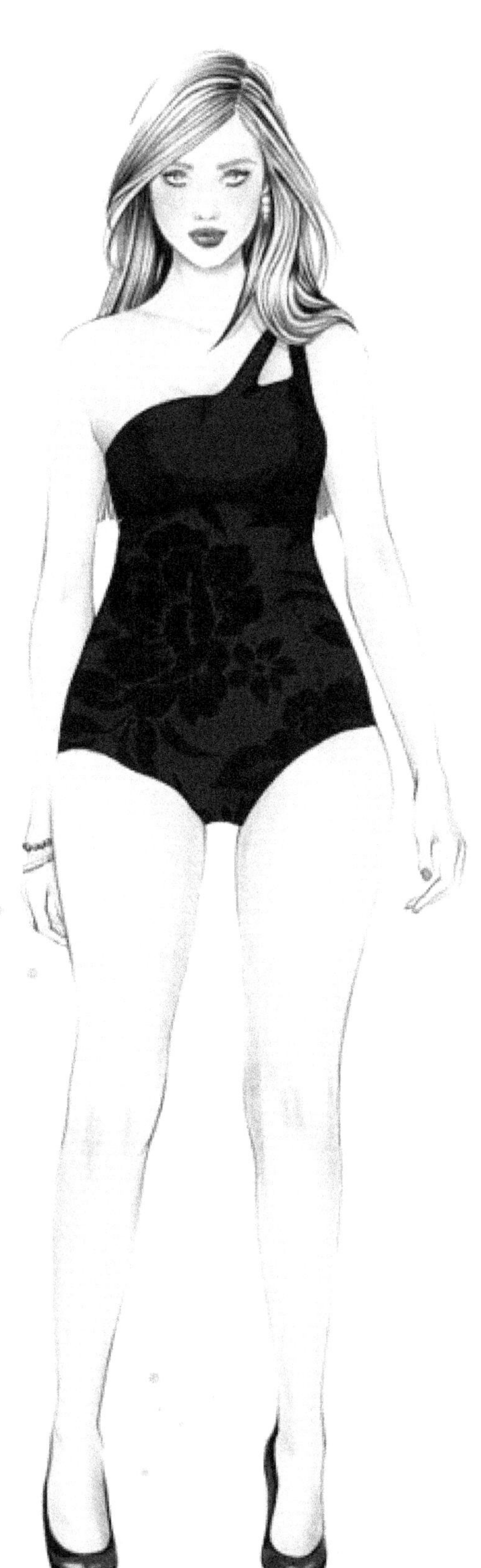

INVERTED TRIANGLE
SHAPE

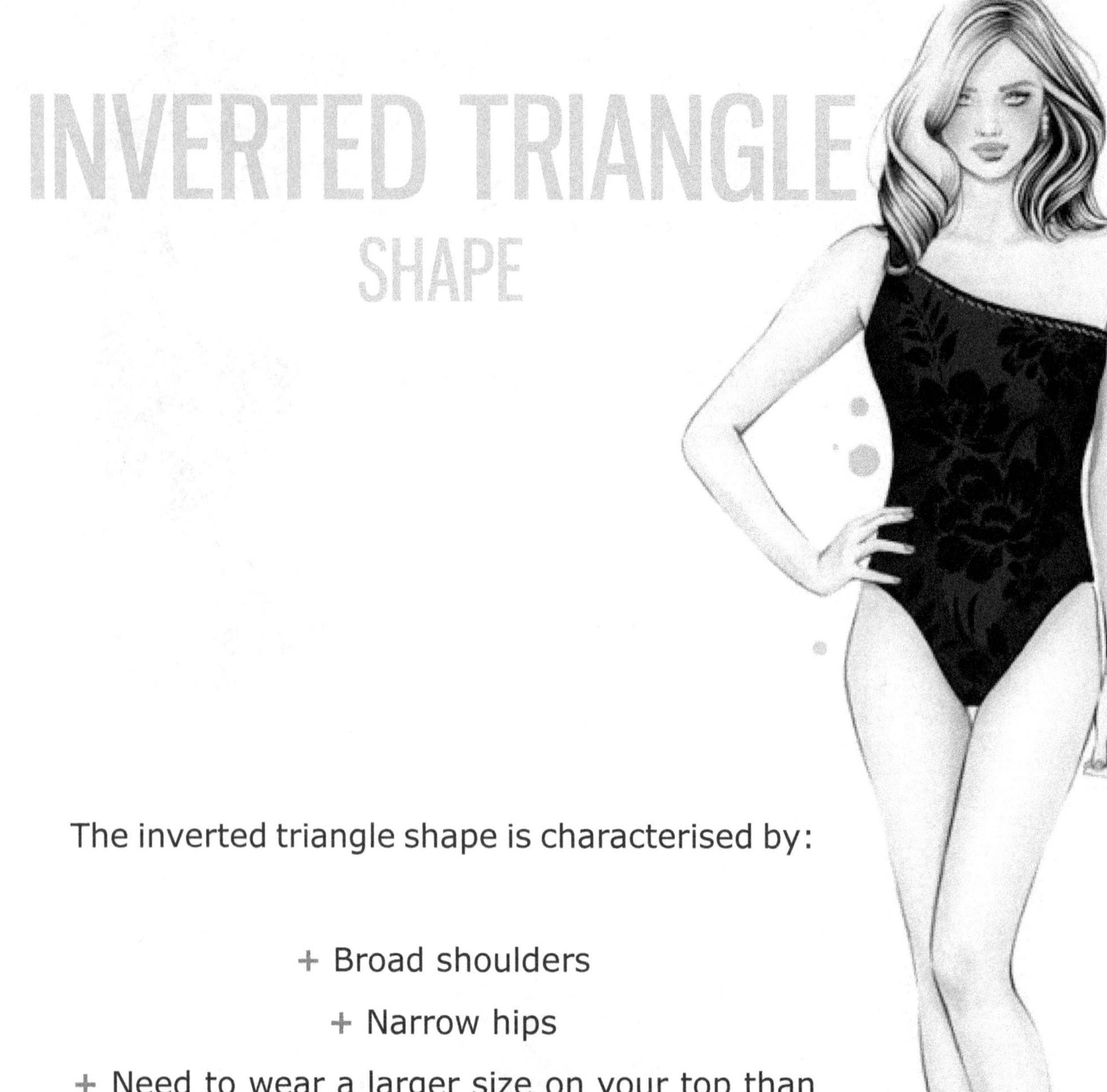

The inverted triangle shape is characterised by:

+ Broad shoulders
+ Narrow hips
+ Need to wear a larger size on your top than your bottom
+ Little definition between your waist and hips
+ Flat bottom

RULER SHAPE

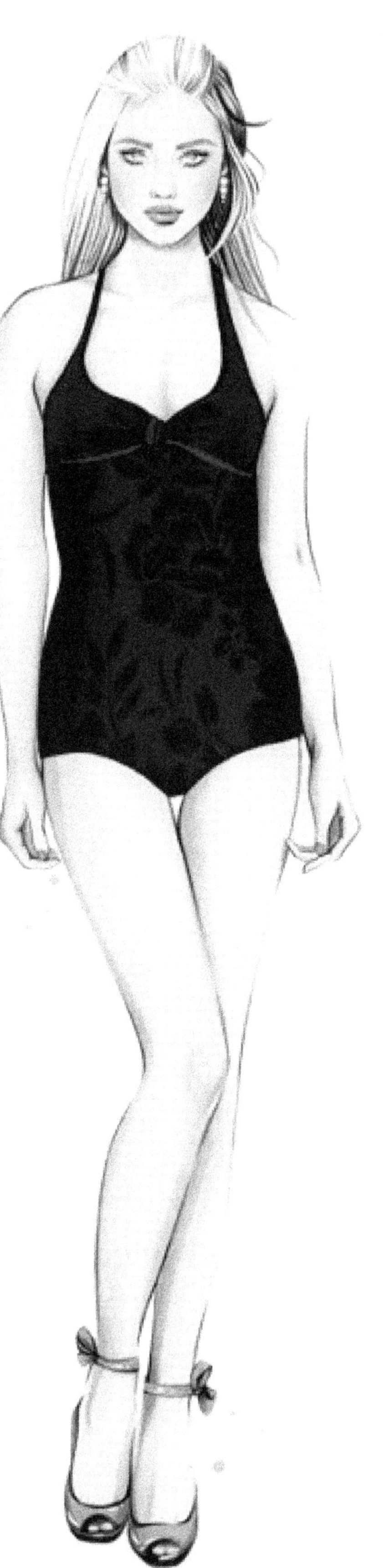

The ruler, aka rectangle, shape is a common female shape that is characterised by:

+ Straight up and down shape
+ No defined shape to the waist
+ Flat hips and bottom
+ Small bust

An apple shape can be difficult to characterise because it is possible that bloating, water retention and hormones are masking your true shape, not to mention that you may be a combination of another shape. In order to determine if you are actually an apple shape, first take a look at the following characteristics:

+ Round and full mid section

+ Undefined waist

+ Rounded shoulders

+ Flattish bottom

+ Narrow hips

+ Gains weight in the belly and breasts

To further clarify, take the circumference measurements of your:

+ Hips + Waist + Bust

If your measurements indicate a larger bust and waist when compared to your hips, such as 39-36-31, you likely do have an apple shape.

APPLE SHAPE

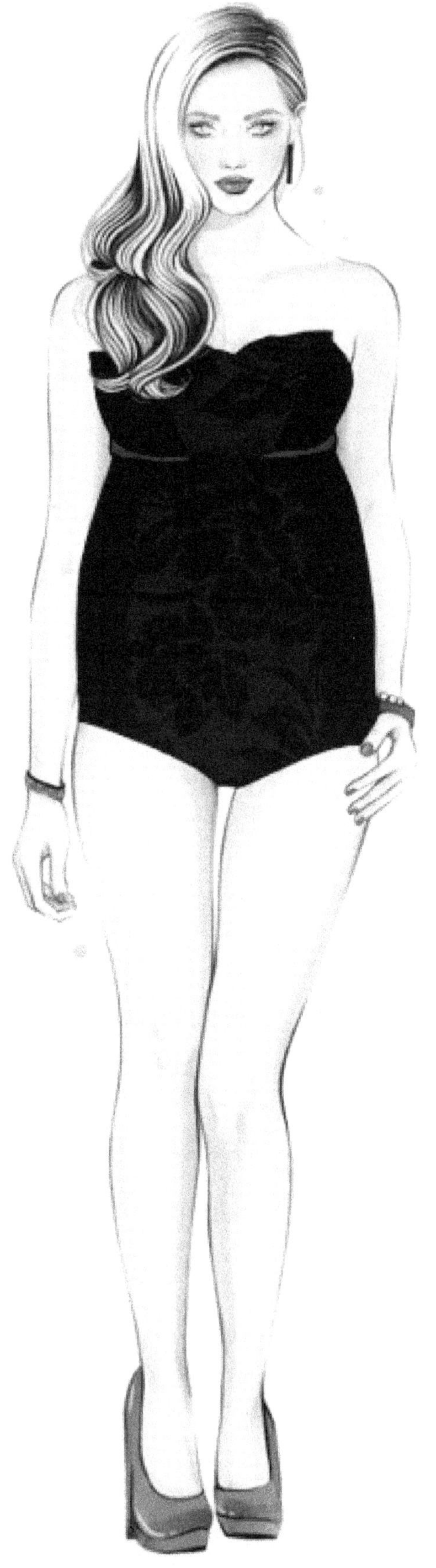

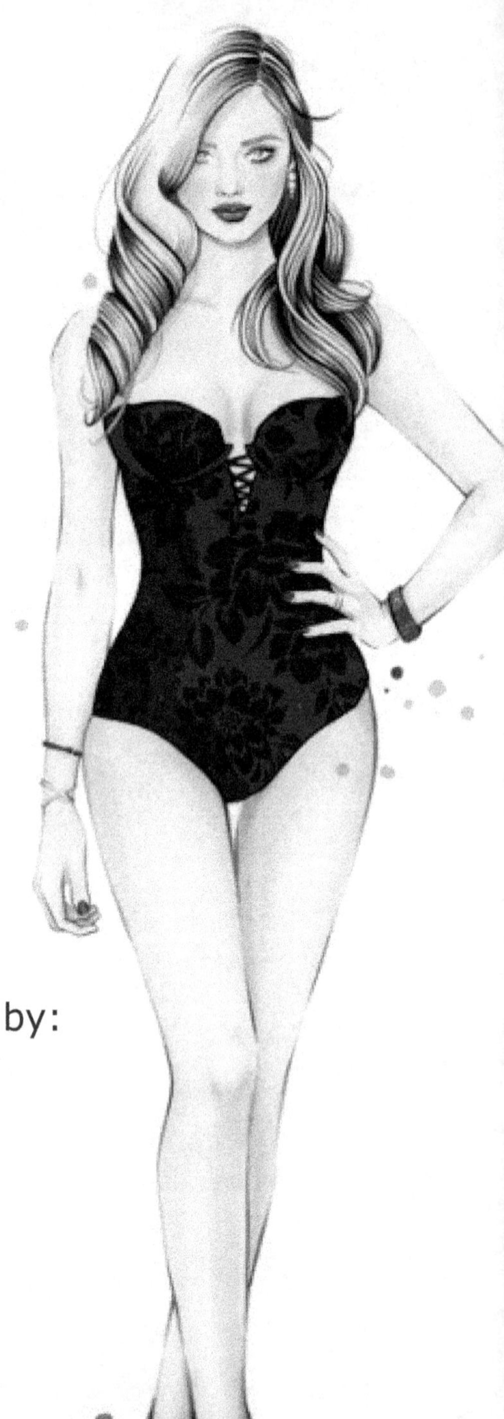

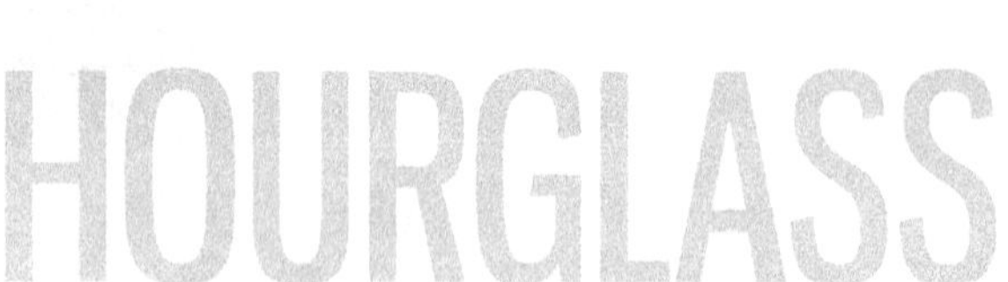

The hourglass shape is characterised by:

+ Curvy, feminine proportions
+ Balanced shoulders and hips
+ A narrow waist
+ Waistbands are often too large
+ Rounded bottom and hips
+ Fuller bust

OVERVIEW

Mainstream fitness programs will tell you to lose weight and train legs often to tone up and shrink your hip dominant pear shape. This advice makes me cringe because this is not how you bring symmetry to your proportions, in fact this approach can exaggerate the imbalance in your proportions. Let me explain.

It is likely that your lower body dominant shape is created by a combination of hip structure and body fat storage, so let's take a look at these.

FAT LOSS

As you may already be aware, body fat cannot be spot reduced. This means that any reductions in body fat will come from all over, including your upper body. Reducing body fat is a great start, and will be included in your program, however, body fat reductions alone will simply result in a smaller pear shape.

To demonstrate this further, please take a look at the following illustration. While this is only a digital representation and your body is obviously unique to you, it is sufficient for the purposes of demonstrating what the underlying structure of a leaned down pear shape could be like.

NUTRITION GUIDELINES

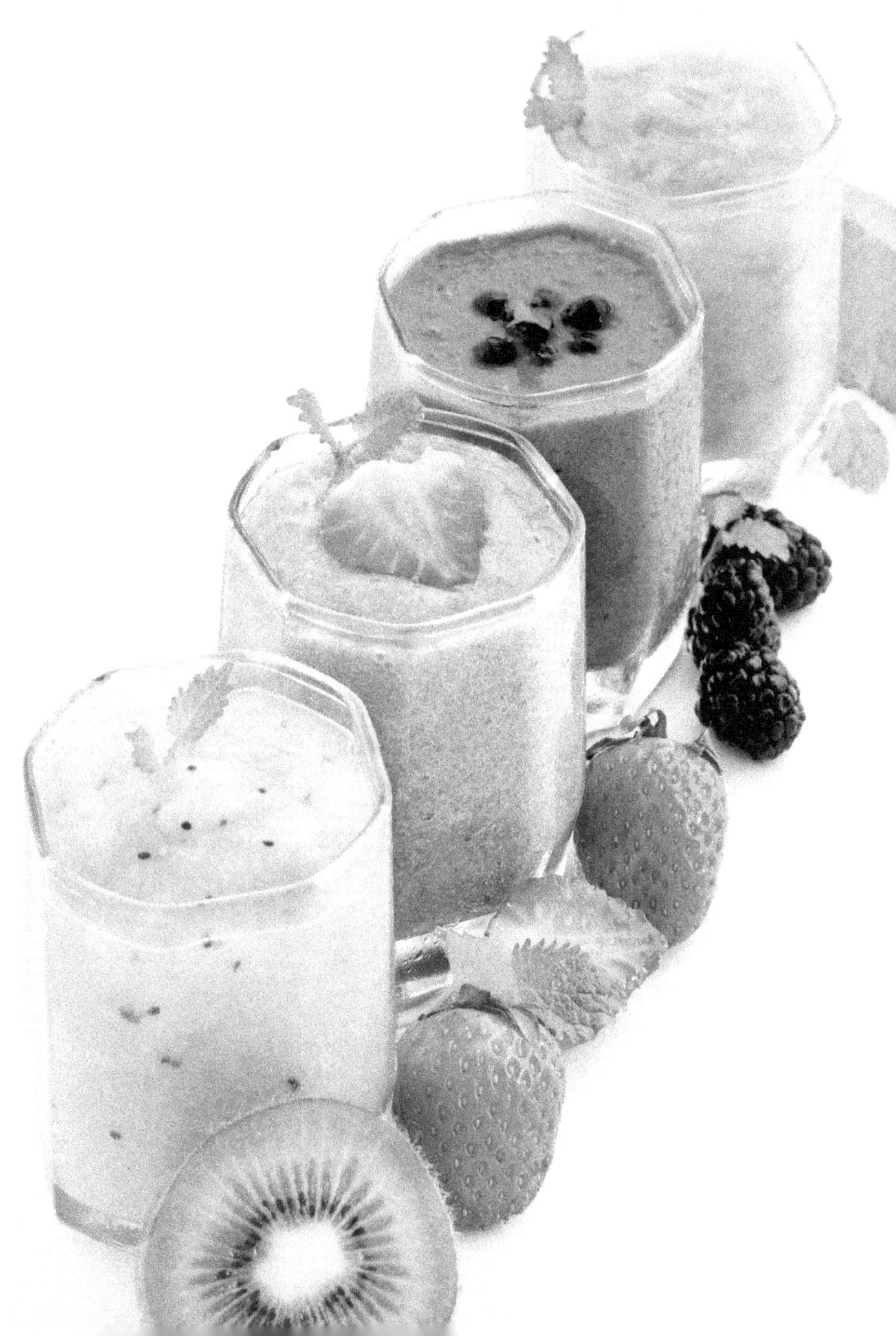

OVERVIEW

This program does not contain any prescribed meal plans because there are so many variables to consider. Plus I don't know what you like or don't like, what you may be intolerant to or what may cause other issues in your life.

For this reason, meal planning will be left to you and I'll simply provide you with the guidance you need to make it effective, along with some sample meal plans and templates to make it understandable and actionable.

CALORIES

Calories are the baseline of any nutrition program, so this is what you'll figure out first. Once you have this number, you'll be able to eat according to your individual body needs, and determine how to factor in your deficit where necessary.

MACROS

Nutrition is not just about calories in and calories out, especially when it comes to body composition goals. More importantly is the ratio and timing of macronutrients. As you are probably aware, the different macronutrients are carbohydrates, protein and fat. Sure, you can lose weight by tracking calories alone, however, your body will look completely different if you also track and optimise your macronutrient profile and timing. Therefore, I'll also provide you with the guideline amounts for the various goals in the program.

TRACKING

In order to keep track of your nutrients, I highly recommend FitDay or MyFitnessPal as this will make your life a lot easier.

When using online calculators, some measurements will be noted as uncooked while others are based on cooked weights. Be sure to input this correctly to get accurate tracking.

CALCULATING

YOUR CALORIES

In order to calculate your calorie requirements, you will use your scale weight as a reference point. This is the only reason your scale weight will be considered. The numbers are simply for the purposes of caloric intake, so don't read too much into those. Remember, muscle weighs more than fat and muscle is good.

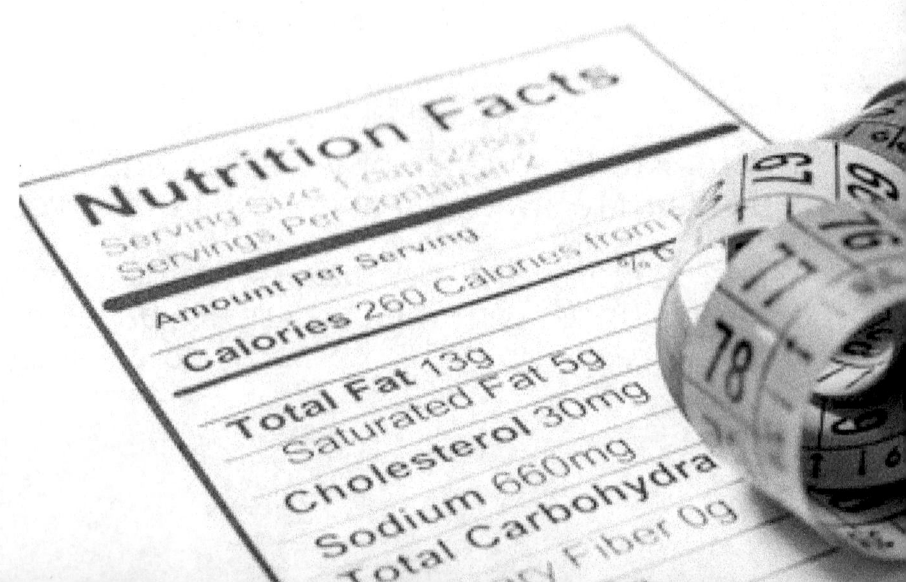

STEP ONE
BASAL METABOLIC RATE (BMR)

First you will need to determine your baseline calories, this is the minimum number of calories your body needs to function while at rest. I've included a handy calculator in your pack, but htere's how it's done manually.

HARRIS-BENEDICT FORMULA

655 + (4.3 x weight in lbs) + (4.7 x height in inches) - (4.7 x age in years) = BMR

EXAMPLE

A female weighing 130lbs, 62 inches high

and 36 years old would calculate:

4.3 x 130 lbs = 559

4.7 x 62 inches = 291.4

4.7 x 36 = 169.2

655 + 559 + 291.4 - 169.2 = BMR 1336.2 calories

STEP TWO
PHYSICAL ACTIVITY LEVEL (PAL)

Next you'll need to factor in your physical activity. This is how many calories you burn through daily activity and will include all activities, from your housework to your job and the gym.

MOSTLY INACTIVE = 1.2

(mainly sitting with little to no exercise)

LIGHTLY ACTIVE = 1.375

(Use this if you are training lightly 3x week)

MODERATELY ACTIVE = 1.55

(Use this if you are training moderately 3-5x week)

VERY ACTIVE = 1.725

(Use this if you are training hard with HIIT's 5x week)

MOSTLY ACTIVE = 1.9

(Use this if you are training hard 5x week with HIIT's and have a physical job)

STEP THREE
TOTAL DAILY ENERGY EXPENDITURE (TDEE)

Finally you'll take your BMR and multiply it by your PAL to discover your TDEE

BMR x PAL = TDEE

Example:

1336.2 **x** 1.55 = TDEE 2071.11 calories

The TDEE number represents how many calories you will need to maintain your current weight. You'll factor in a deficit or surplus based on this number as your maintenance point.

This formula is one of the most accurate methods of calculating your energy needs, however, these numbers are subject to a little trial and error due to activity and exertion levels varying from person to person. Adjust this multiplier if necessary to find what works for you.

TRIM PHASE
ADJUSTMENTS

During the Trim phase when fat burning is your goal, you'll naturally be eating below your maintenance TDEE calories. Now, because we are all unique, with varying degrees of motivation and starting points, and unique daily challenges, I don't believe in giving a rigid one size fits all number. Rather, I like to provide two options that you can choose from according to how fast you feel you want to progress and how much sacrifice you are willing to make daily. You will still make great progress with either option, however, one will be slightly steadier than the other. These choices are:

CONSERVATIVE DEFICIT = 15-20%
MODERATE DEFICIT = 20-25%

Let's take a look at those in turn.

15-20%
CONSERVATIVE CALORIE DEFICIT

Within this conservative deficit range, you'll:

PRESERVE AND GROW MUSCLE BETTER

+ BUT FAT LOSS WILL BE SLOWER

ENJOY LIFE THAT LITTLE BIT MORE

+ WHILE STILL DROPPING BODY FAT

A smaller deficit may suit you better if:

+ You find yourself getting overly hungry
+ You have an active job which requires higher amounts of energy
+ You find it difficult to stick to a higher restriction
+ You're happy to focus more on overall composition goals

20-25%

MODERATE CALORIE DEFICIT

Within this moderate deficit range, you'll:

REDUCE BODY FAT FASTER

+ BUT YOUR MUSCLE GROWTH WILL BE SLOWER

YOU'LL BE MORE RESTRICTED

+ BUT FAT LOSS WILL BE FASTER

A moderate deficit may suit you better if:

+ You are highly motivated and okay with a higher restriction
+ You have a desk job that requires little exertion

STAGGER
YOUR CALORIE INTAKE

There are two ways I like to stagger my calories to keep things changing and to fit them into my lifestyle. These are:

On a day to day basis, you may stagger your calories so that on training days your intake is higher than those on rest days. This is known as cycling. We use this method so that your energy is partitioned when it will be used. Using the 20-25 deficit range, here is an example of how this works:

TRAINING DAYS = LOWER DEFICIT (e.g 20%)

NON-TRAINING DAYS = HIGHER DEFICIT (e.g 25%)

You can even use a weekly rotation, using a stricter 20-25% for 3 weeks and then taking a lighter 15-20% for the fourth. Or if you have a trip coming up that you want to be more social for, you can use the higher deficit until the trip and then lower the deficit during without sabotaging your progress. Whatever works for you. This is a lifestyle, not a restrictive diet.

SCULPT PHASE
ADJUSTMENTS

During the Sculpt phase when your body is much leaner and muscle growth is top priority, you'll remain at your maintenance level or in a slight surplus of 10% above maintenance this is because muscle will only grow with a sufficient intake of calories.

You can build muscles while in a caloric deficit, but it is extremely difficult to do. As long as your activity intensity is strong, the additional calories you ingest will be properly proportioned to your muscles, and you cal always drop back to the Trim phase if you want to rein in any fat gains. Trust the process.

CONSERVATIVE SURPLUS = 10% or MAINTENANCE CALORIES

FIND WHAT
WORKS FOR YOU

You need to use a starting point to see how your body responds, and then make any adjustments from there. Therefore I would suggest starting out on the 15-20% range and seeing how you get on. The reason I suggest the lower count is because why would you cut more food out than is necessary? However, this is totally your choice and just my opinion. Once you have done this for a week, you can decide whether a higher deficit is necessary. In order for this to be accurate, you'll need to stick to the calorie intake as closely as possible.

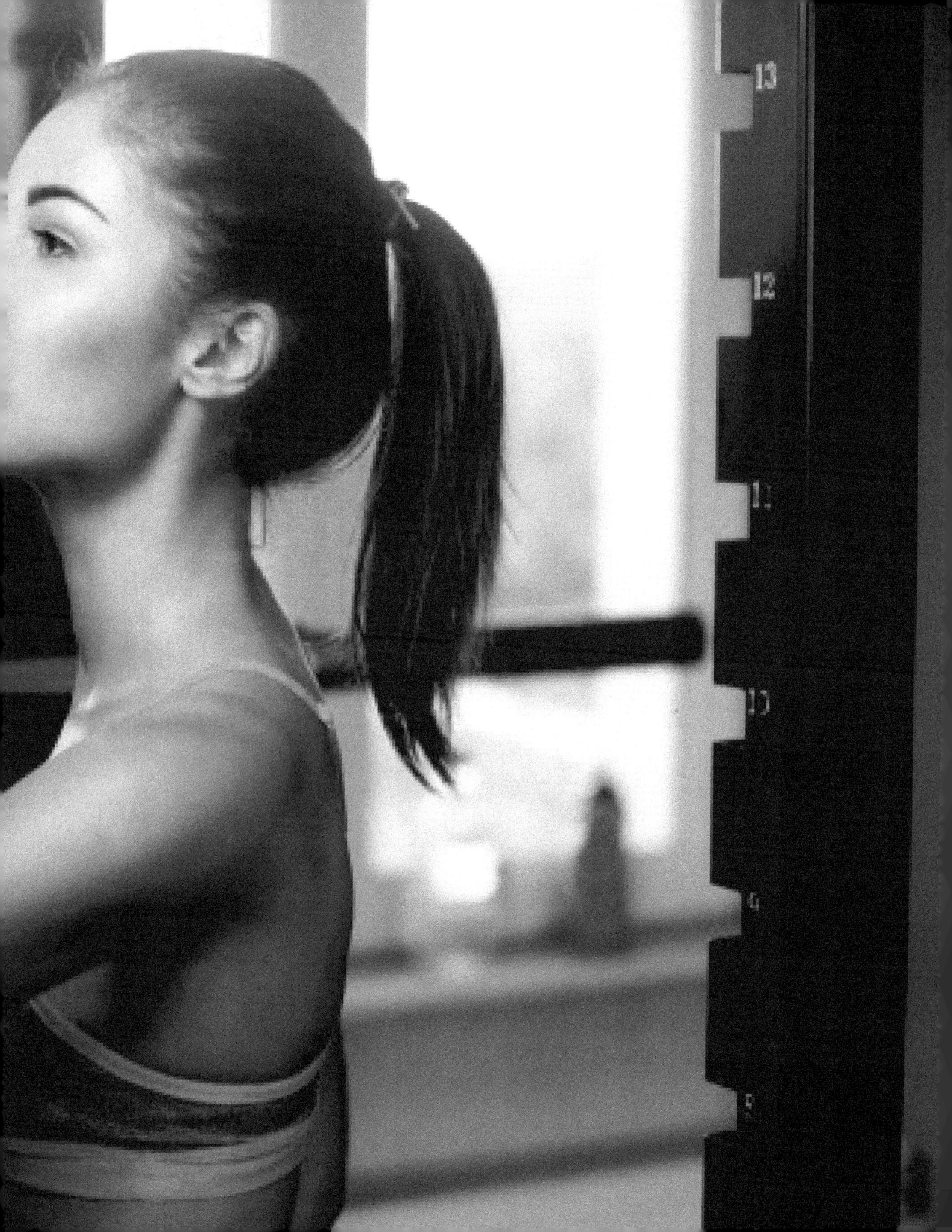

13
12
11

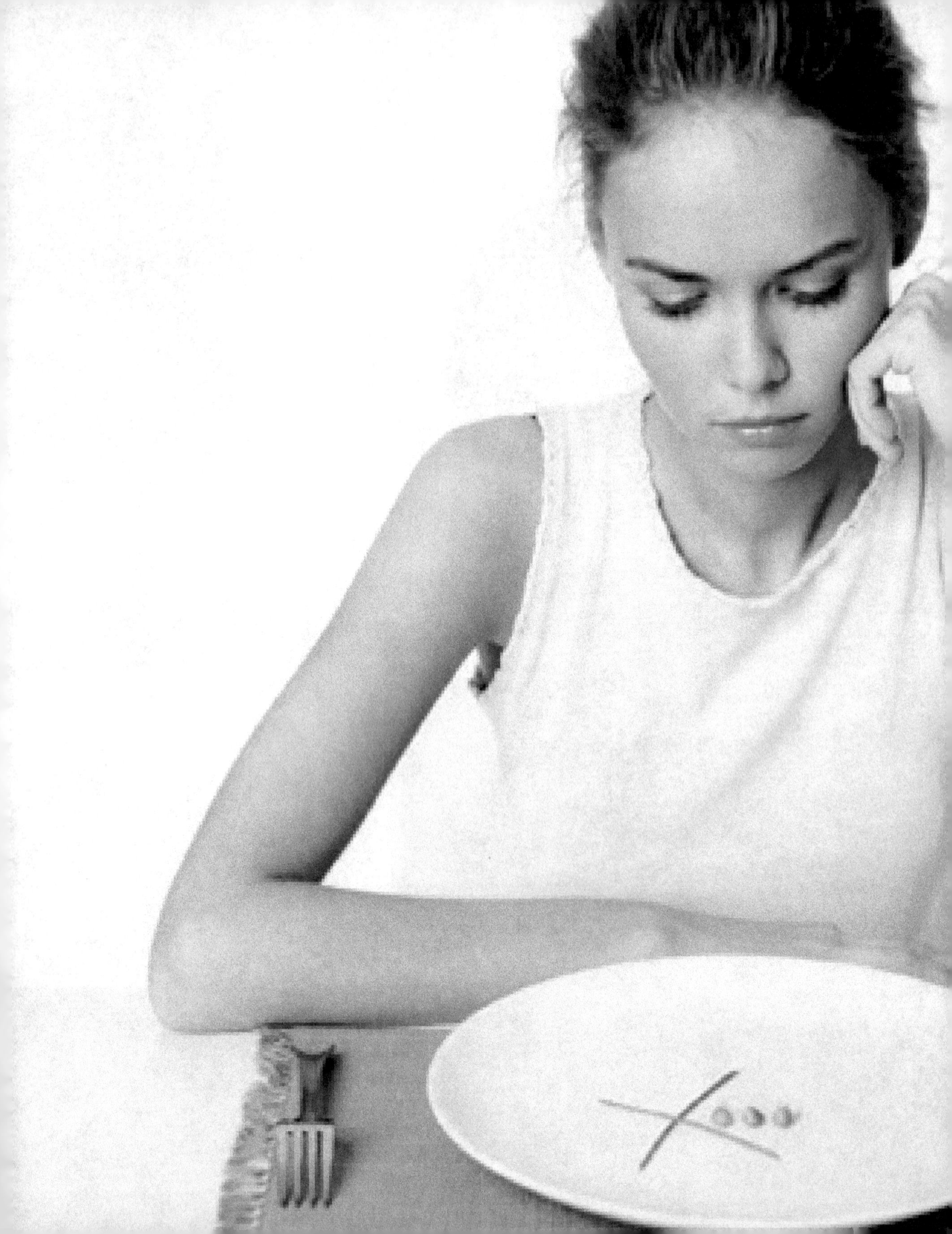

RECALCULATE
REGULARLY

As you get leaner, your calorie intake will need to reduce in line with your new weight. Likewise if you activity level or intensity changes, you will also need to adjust accordingly. Therefore please recalculate your calorie requirements should your weight or activity change significantly.

To make life simpler and keep calorie restrictions pain free, I reduce my daily calorie intake by 30 calorie increments each week that goes by. This may not sound a lot, but over 12 weeks that adds up to 330 calories removed from your total daily allowance.

Therefore, someone starting off on 1800 calories would have 1770 the following week, 1740 the next, 1710 the next and so on. Ending up with 1470 after 12 weeks.

TIMING YOUR MEALS

You may have heard that eating smaller and more frequent meals throughout the day raises you metabolism and helps you lose more weight. Here's the thing. Fat loss or gain is dependent on energy balance, aka calories in vs calories out. It has nothing to do with how many meals you have.

Many studies have been conducted that show eating smaller and more frequent meals actually has little bearing on fat loss. In fact, it is shown that larger meals cause larger metabolic spikes than do smaller one's and those spikes last longer too. It is true that eating little and often makes your body work harder to break down a continual flow of food, however, this isn't necessarily a good thing for your organs.

The second reasoning behind little and often is appetite suppression, however, this too has been shown to differ from person to person so also remains inconclusive. As a matter of fact, smaller portion sizes, when your calorie requirements are small to begin with, can leave you feeling deprived and unfulfilled. Think about 1500 calories divided over 6 meals, that's 250 calories per meal. Would you be satisfied with that?

There is another group in favour of smaller meals that show a positive benefit on controlling blood sugar levels, but again the integrity of this result has been questioned. So, all in all, the bottom line is that there's no consensus on which is better than the other. Ultimately, whether you eat 3 meals a day, 3 meals an 2 snacks or even 6 is entirely your choice and what you find suits you and your lifestyle. If you find eating 3 meals a day is most satisfying and fits in with your lifestyle, then by all means continue to use that principle.

LATE NIGHT EATING

A friend of mine recently messaged me late in the evening in a panic. Her work had gone on later than expected and she had arrived home with one meal still left to consume. She was panicking because it was late and she feared late night eating. Her question was, should I miss this meal and just go to bed hungry or eat it and risk putting on weight. I once had the same fear so I can completely relate, however, this is a fallacy.

As mentioned above, meal timing isn't an important factor, energy balance is. In fact, missing a meal and being too far under your daily calorie requirements has more drastic consequences than the time you eat your meal, so I urge you never miss a meal just because it is late in the day.

In fact, when in this situation, the best course of action is to consume a slow digesting protein source, such as a casein shake or some cottage cheese, along with some fats. This will fill the gap, bring your calories up to balance and will aid in the recovery of your muscles while you sleep. It's a win win.

While regularity of food and late night eating isn't the problem they are made out to be, nutrient timing is a tool that can be beneficial for the purposes of optimising body composition. Let's take a look at these in turn.

CALCULATING MACROS

There are 3 types of macronutrients that are essential to the body. They are proteins, carbohydrates and fats. Every food falls into one of these categories, and their classification is determined by which macronutrient is dominant. For example, 100 grams of Quinoa contains 68.9g of carbs, 13.1g of protein and 5.8g of fat. Because the dominant macronutrient is carbohydrates, Quinoa is categorised as a carbohydrate, even though it contains traces of the other macronutrients.

The key thing to remember is that the weight of the food doesn't equal the weight of the macronutrient (unless the food is 100% a certain macro, like sugar, or coconut oil).

For example, if your protein allowance is 35g per meal, to obtain 35g of protein from pork tenderloin, you will need 135g of pork tenderloin. This is calculated using the following equation:

100 ÷ the amount of protein per 100g x your allowance

So for Chicken breast, turkey breast or salmon:

100 ÷ 25 = 4

4 x 35 = 140

If this seems a little confusing, check out MyFitnessPal or FitDay. This will make calculations a breeze and leave you to enjoy life.

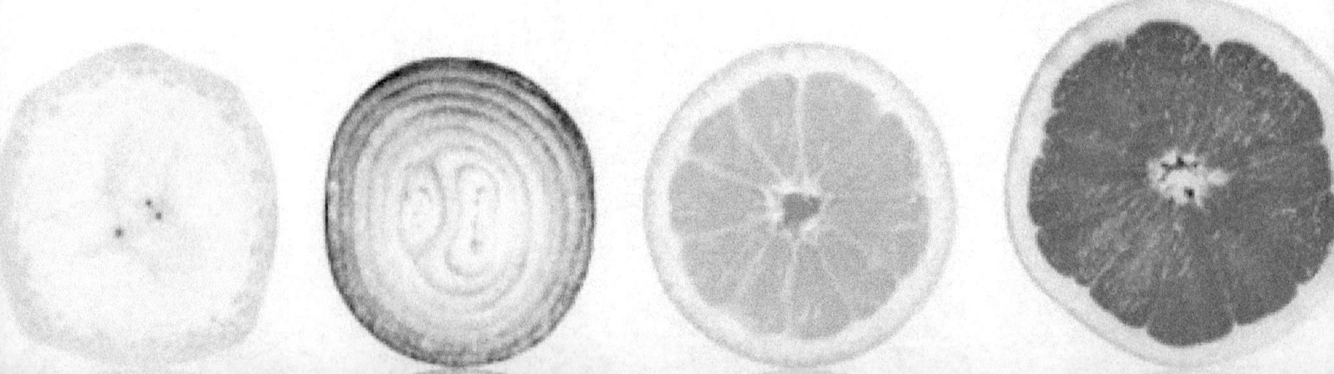

CARBOHYDRATES

Carbohydrates turn to glucose in the body and glucose is the body's preferred source of energy.

You'll want to limit your intake of processed carbs and those high on the glycemic index, such as white bread, white pasta and white rice, as well as refined sugars, which is essentially anything ending in -ose on a packet such as sucrose, fructose, dextrose and glucose. These all produce large glucose spikes and increase demands on your body to produce insulin.

Over production of insulin can lead to abdominal fat, so should be kept to the minimum. After training is the only time high GI carbs are necessary. For meals that not immediately after training, stick to lower GI carbs such as sweet potato, brown rice, and wholegrain pasta.

1g CARBS = 4 CALORIES

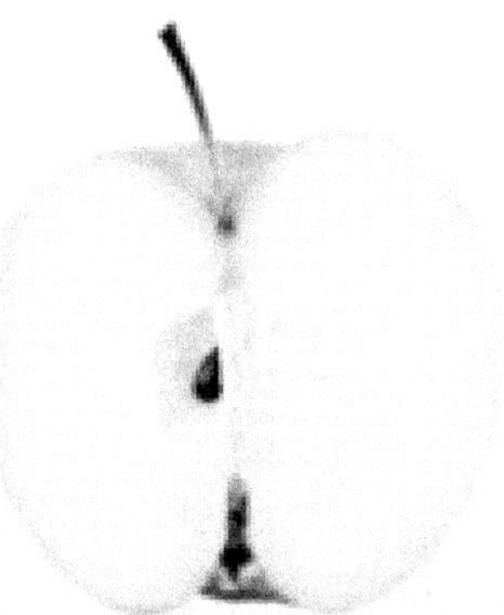
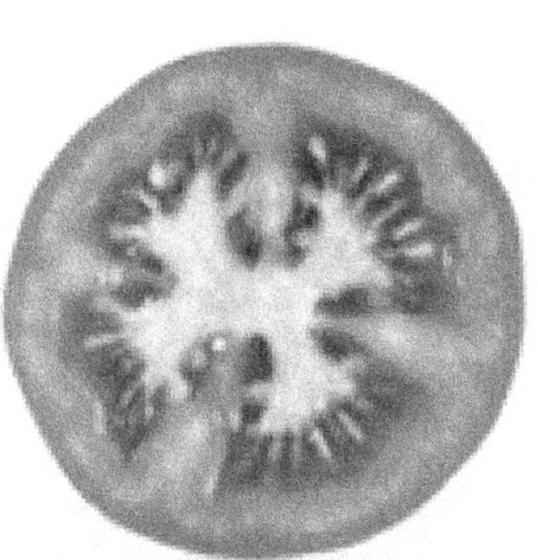
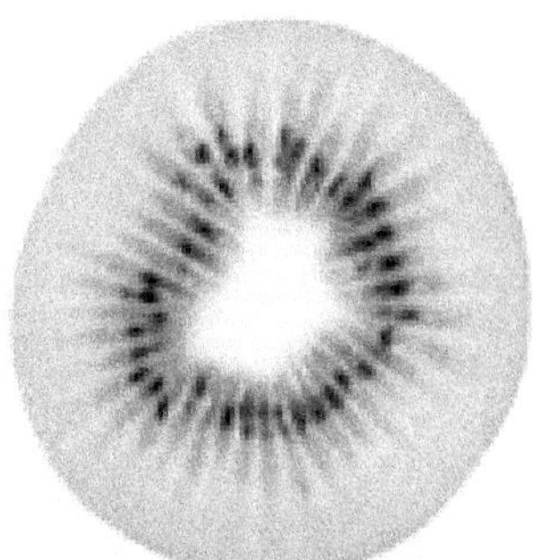
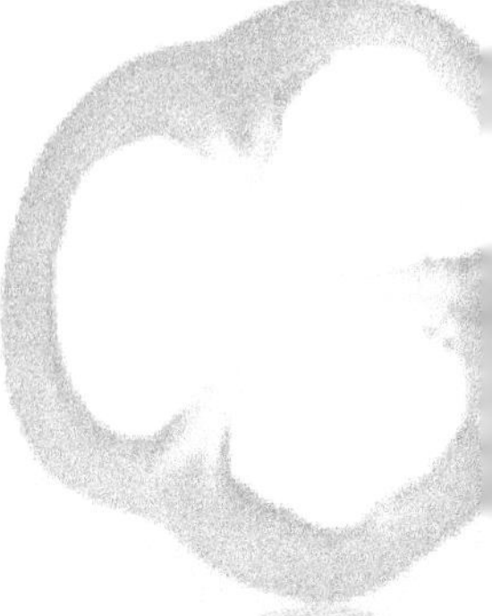

MIND THE WHEAT

Wheat has a lot of controversy associated with it, particularly as many people are intolerant to the gluten in wheat. If you feel the need, you can eliminate wheat from your diet and see if it has a positive impact.

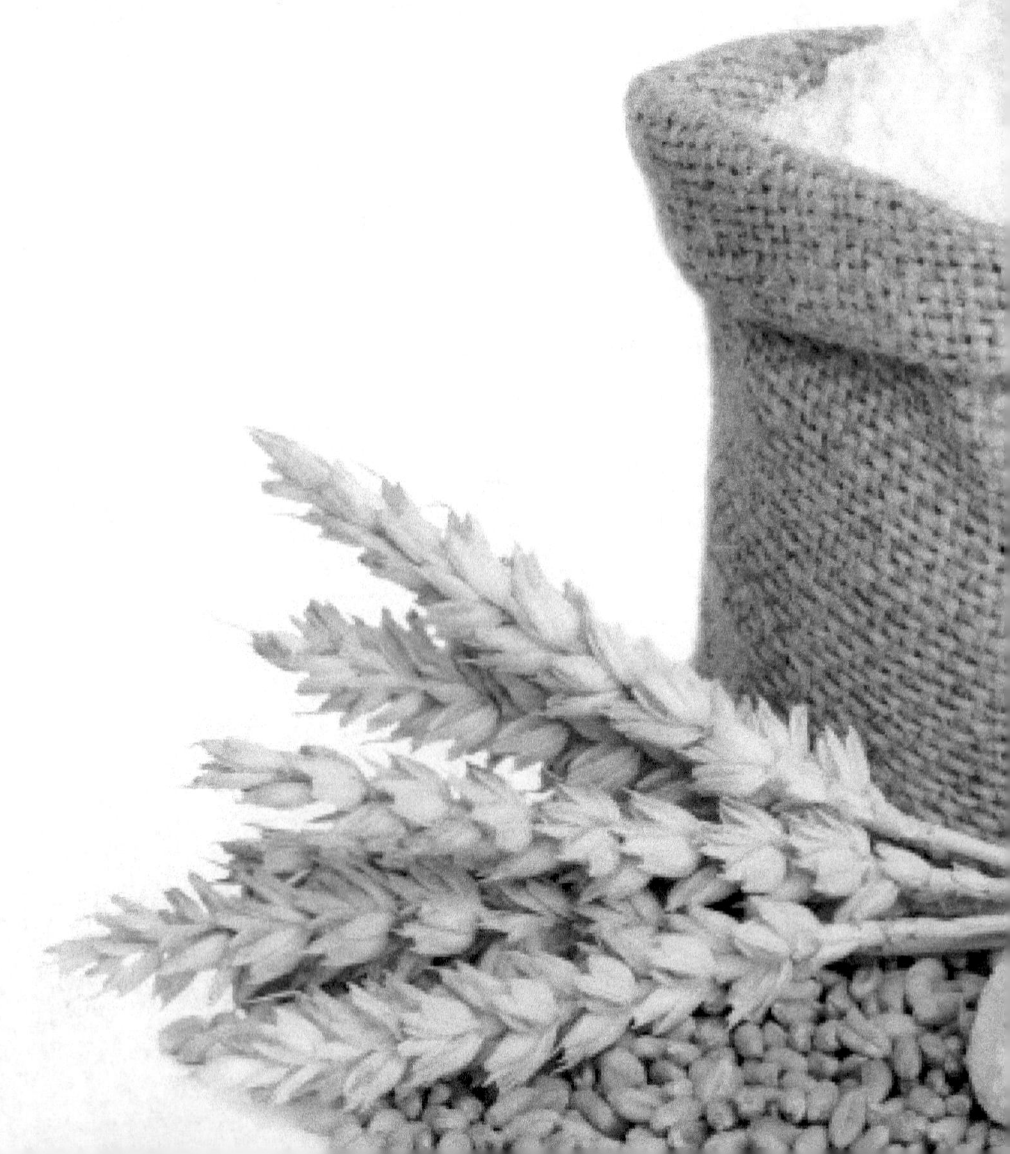

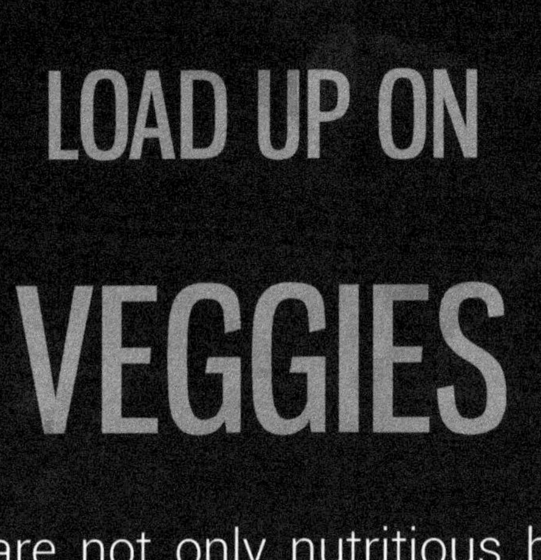

LOAD UP ON VEGGIES

Vegetables are not only nutritious but are also great sources of fibre. They are low in calories and very filling. Some vegetables are higher GI such as sweetcorn, peas and carrots, while others are lower GI such as broccoli, asparagus and cabbage. Try sticking to low GI veggies as much as possible but, more importantly, get as many different colour vegetables into your meals as possible.

EAT AT LEAST TWO PORTIONS PER MEAL

TIMING YOUR CARBS

Timing of your carb intake is very important.

As we covered in a previous section, when you eat carbohydrates, they are digested and turned into glucose. Insulin is released in response to glucose and it's job is to shuttle the glucose into your muscle or fat cells for energy or storage.

First thing in the morning, your muscle cells are generally not receptive, so **carbohydrates for breakfast will likely partition those nutrients to your fat stores rather than into your muscles.** This is also the case on rest days when you are mostly sedentary. Conversely, after exercising at a high intensity or weight training, your muscle glycogen stores become depleted, therefore making your muscle cells highly receptive. This is the best time to introduce carbs into your meal plan.

For this reason, I suggest a method referred to as carb cycling.

EAT CARBS IMMEDIATELY AFTER TRAINING

After training, muscles are primed for carbs, so use this time to increase your intake. This is also the best time to have higher GI simple carbs because you'll want the insulin spike to shuttle protein to your muscle cells quickly. I suggest you consume 1/4 of your daily allowance within 30 minutes of training.

Dextrose powder is fast absorbed and is a ideal carb supplement for post exercise, fruit and carbs are a little slower to release but are also good choices.

AVOID CARBS BEFORE BED

With the absence of carbs before bed, you body can turn to fat stores during the extended hours of sleep rather than breaking down those carbs for it's fuel

PROTEIN

Protein is the most important macronutrient. Protein is essential for cellular growth and repair in all parts of the body. Protein is made up of amino acids. 12 of those are manufactured by the body and 9 must be obtained by food. These 9 are called essential amino acids. Any food item which contains all 9 is referred to as a complete protein. Any food that doesn't contain all 9 are incomplete proteins.

Complete proteins include animal sources, such as red meat, poultry, fish, eggs, and dairy. You'll also find that protein powder and BCAA supplements are also complete. Incomplete sources include peas, beans, lentils, whole grains, nuts, and seeds. As a vegetarian, you'll need to combine two incomplete proteins or use a soybean based protein powder.

1g PROTEIN = 4 CALORIES

CARB COUNTS

CARB SOURCE	CARB PER 100G
Mung Beans	63g
Raw Lentils	60g
Wheatgerm	52g
Quinoa	23g
Brown Rice	23g
Sweet Potato	23g
Boiled Lentils	20g
Butternut Squash	12g

PROTEIN
TIMING GUIDELINES

Protein is the most important macronutrient as far as body composition goes, and there are several times throughout the day where they are particularly important. These are:

IMMEDIATELY AFTER TRAINING

To maximise recovery after training, drink a whey protein shake and some BCAA's immediately following your training. When combined with your carbs, these will enhance recovery and promote muscle building. You could also add a small amount of casein whey to your shake to prolong those effects.

BEFORE FASTED CARDIO

Similar to above, when your body is in a fasted state and in the absence of protein, energy is more likely to be taken from breaking down muscle fibres to fuel your cardio. Drinking a BCAA supplement before fasted training will help to preserve muscles and turn your body to using fat for fuel instead. Yeah, BCAA supplements are pretty awesome.

BEFORE CARBS

Protein slows down the absorption rate of carbs, which also lowers the release of insulin, not to mention that it will be the protein that is shuttled to your muscles when the insulin is released. Therefore, always eat some protein before tucking into your carbs.

UPON WAKING

After your body has fasted overnight, you'll want to get protein into your system as quickly as possible to avoid potential breakdown of muscle fibres. Whole food proteins will take too long to break down, so this is where a BCAA supplement is ideal. It's fast releasing and contains minimal calories.

BEFORE BED

Ingesting a slow releasing protein before bed, such as casein whey or cottage cheese, can help prevent muscle breakdown during your sleeping hours. This is because your body will break down the amino acids in the protein, rather than your muscle fibers.

KEEP IT EVEN

Your body can only synthesise a certain amount of protein at one time. This has been said to be around 20g. In addition, your body needs a regular and constant flow of protein to keep it from burning muscle fibres, therefore, spread your protein intake as evenly as possible, taking into account the guidelines set out above.

PROTEIN COUNTS

PROTEIN SOURCE	PROTEIN PER 100G
Pork Tenderloin	26g
Chicken Breast	25g
Turkey Breast	25g
Salmon	25g
Trout	24g
Venison	24g
Lean Turkey Breast Mince	23g
Lean Chicken Breast Mince	23g
Beef Steak	23g
Lean ground beef mince	23g
Wild Boar	22g
White Fish	20g
Haddock	19g
Mackerel	19g
Prawns	15g
Eggs	13g

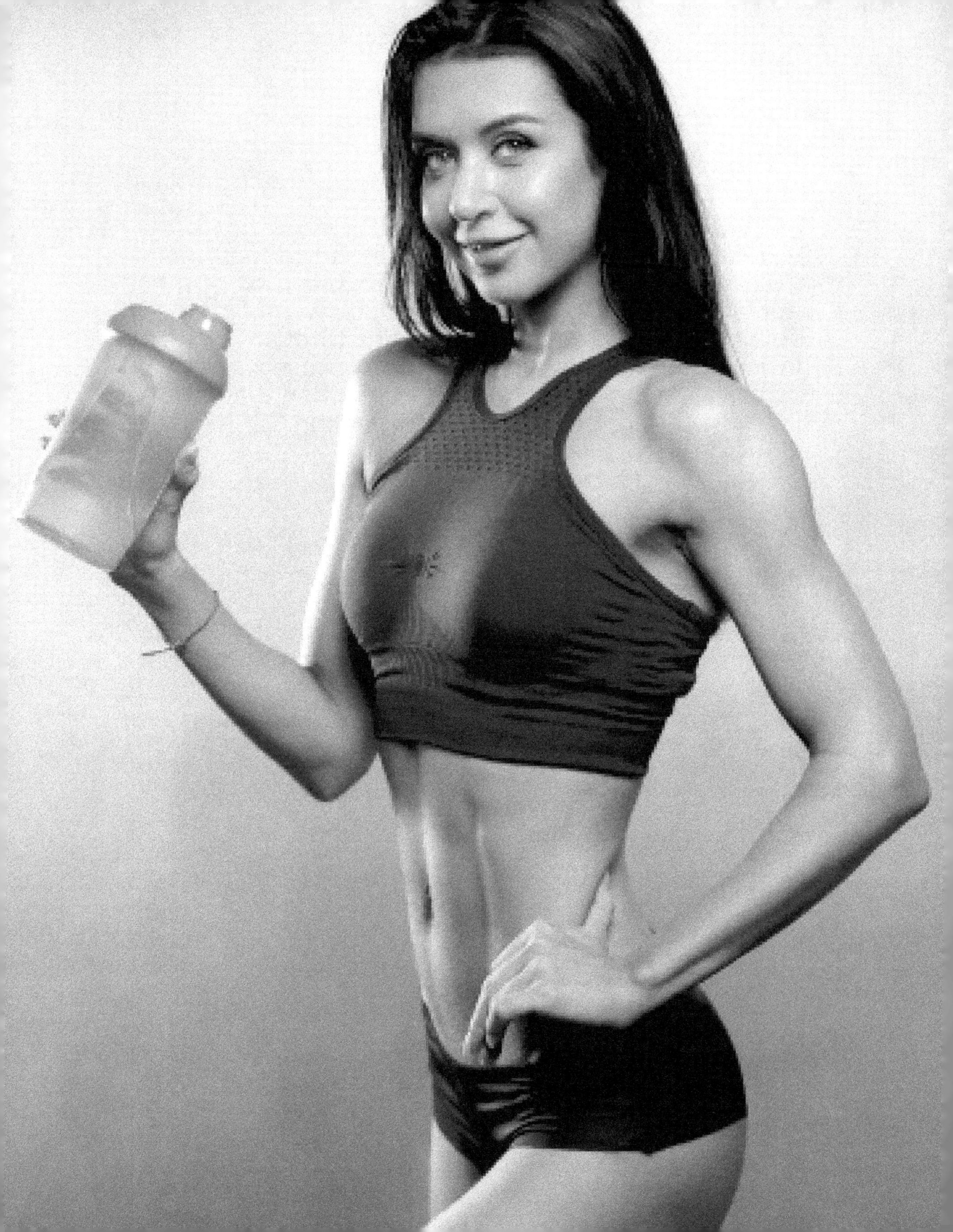

DIETARY FATS

At 9 calories per 1 gram of fat, fat is the most dense macronutrient of all, which is why it has a bit of a bad reputation. Sure too much can cause weight gain and it's high density can make it easier to over consume, however, too much of any macro can cause weight gain so this is not limited to fat. Not to mention that fats are highly satiating, so will keep you feeling full for much longer.

Fats are vital for many body functions, including cellular repair, hormone function and lubrication of the joints. Not to mention great for the condition of your skin and hair. Good fats such as those found in oily fish, red meat, nuts, seeds, dairy, avocados, coconut and olive oil should be used within your program according to the macro range set. Avoid trans fats, but don't fear good healthy fats.

1g FAT = 9 CALORIES

FAT TIMING

There are two times in the day where it is most beneficial to ingest your fats, these are at breakfast and before bed.

AT BREAKFAST

Fats are highly satiating, so having those at breakfast, where you'll now be eliminating carbs, will keep you feeling full for longer and reduce the need for any additional snacking. Furthermore, the absence of carbs will limit the potential for an insulin spike to send those fats to storage.

AVOID AFTER EXERCISE

Fats after exercise is off limits. Including fats at this time will decrease the effectiveness of your post exercise meal. Slowing down this post exercise meal will make it more likely that the meal will be siphoned into fat stores.

BEFORE BED

Fats alongside your casein protein before bed will slow the digestion rate of the protein even further, preventing muscle breakdown for even longer.

FAT COUNTS

FAT SOURCE	FAT PER 100G
Coconut Oil	100g
MCT Oil	93g
Extra Virgin Olive Oil	91g
Macadamia Nuts	75g
Brazil Nuts	68g
Walnuts	68g
Almonds	50g
Flaxseeds	46g
Cashews	44g
Peanuts	44g
Chia Seeds	31g
Avocados	19g

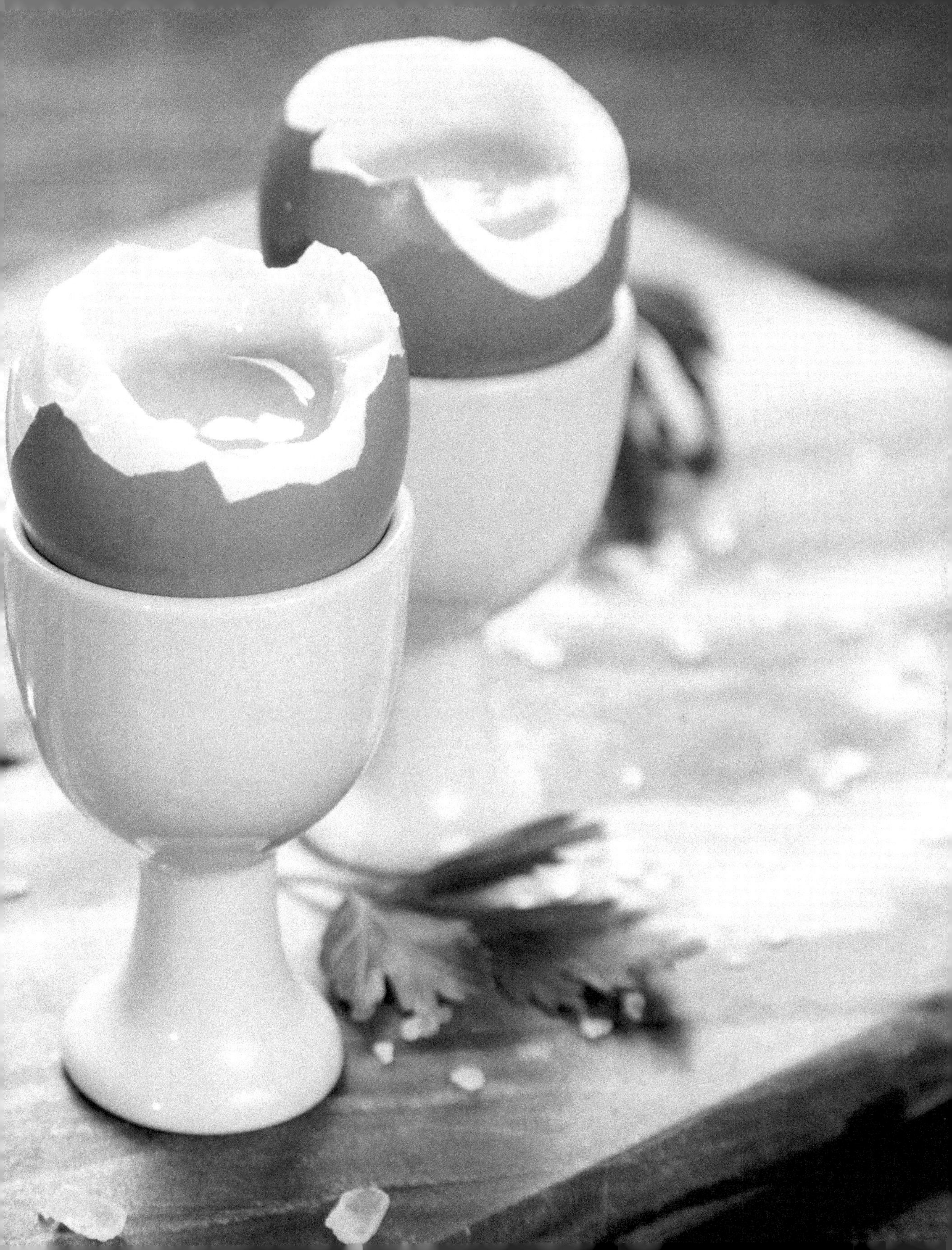

ECTOMORPHS

Ectomorphs have fast and efficient metabolisms, and therefore tend to be naturally slim and wiry.

As an ectomorph, you're already prone to being slim due to your fast metabolism, so you'll want to skip the Trim phase and launch full steam ahead into the Sculpt phase in order to begin building out the curves of your petite frame.

As you likely will experience difficulties gaining any sort of weight and developing your muscles, I suggest a 10% calorie surplus on both training and non-training days, and keeping your carbohydrates higher than those suggested in the program, say 55% and see how you get on with that. To help with the muscle building process, mix BCAA's with some honey and drink it during your training.

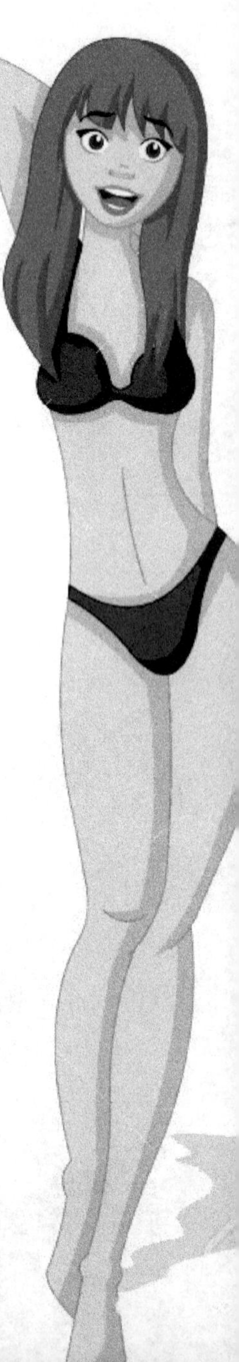

TRAINING & REST DAYS = 10% CALORIE SURPLUS

CARBS 55% / PROTEIN 25% / FAT 20%

ENDOMORPHS

Endomorphs have a sluggish metabolism so gain weight easily and, therefore, tend to appear soft and curvy.

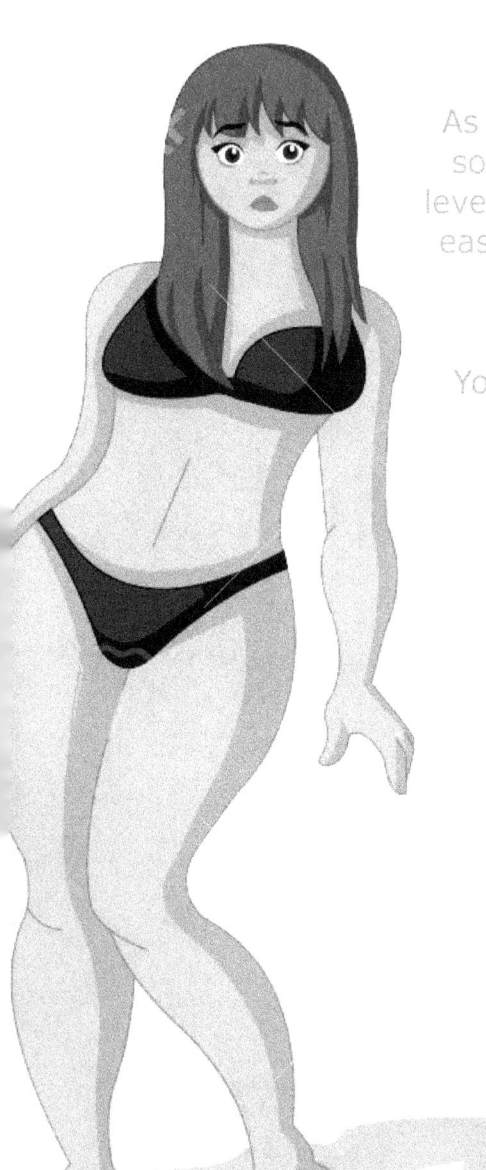

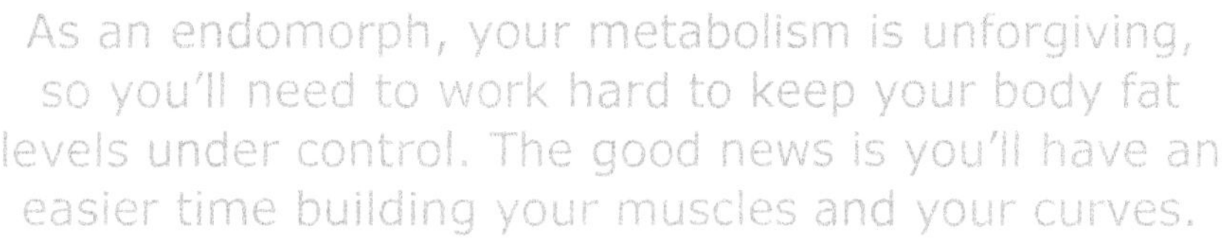

As an endomorph, your metabolism is unforgiving, so you'll need to work hard to keep your body fat levels under control. The good news is you'll have an easier time building your muscles and your curves.

You'll want to steer clear of high GI carbs to limit your insulin spikes as much as possible.

SCULPT PHASE

TRAINING DAYS = EAT MAINTENANCE CALORIES

REST DAYS = 10% CALORIE DEFICIT

CARBS 25% / PROTEIN 35% / FAT 40%

TRIM PHASE

TRAINING DAYS = 20% CALORIE DEFICIT

REST DAYS = 25% CALORIE DEFICIT

VEGGIE CARBS 25% / PROTEIN 35% / FAT 40%

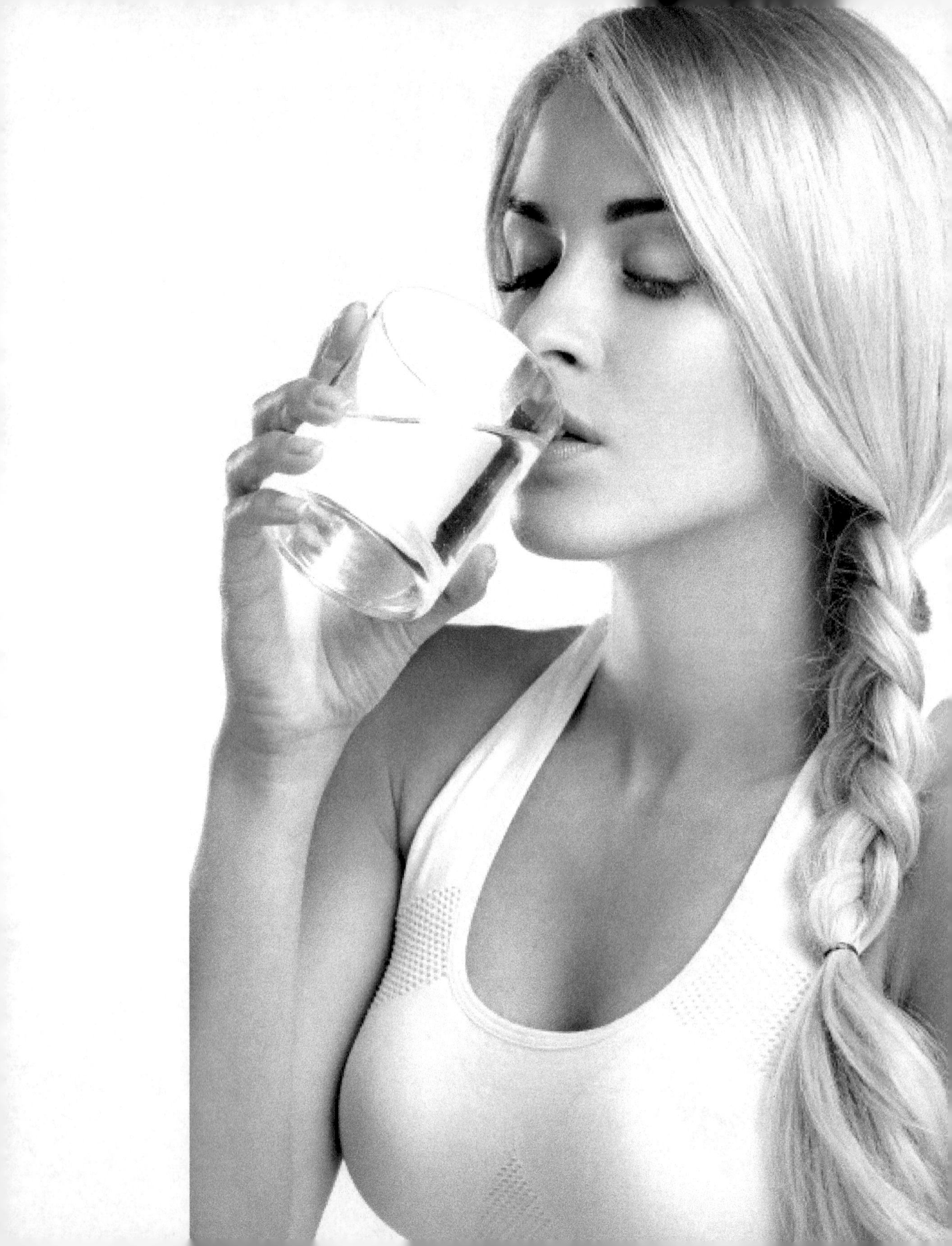

HYDRATION

Water is essential for metabolising stored fat for energy. If your water intake is insufficient, you kidneys becomes dehydrated and your liver will not function optimally to break down fat. Dehydration also leads to constipation, fluid retention and bloating, so it is important to avoid dehydration at all costs.

As a side benefit, water is great for suppressing appetite and keeping you full between meals. You'll find your performance is better when properly hydrated.

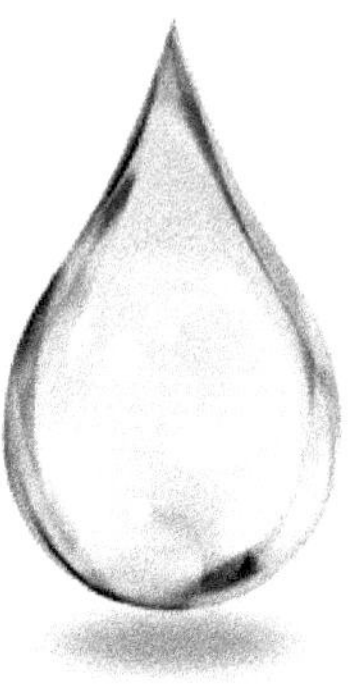

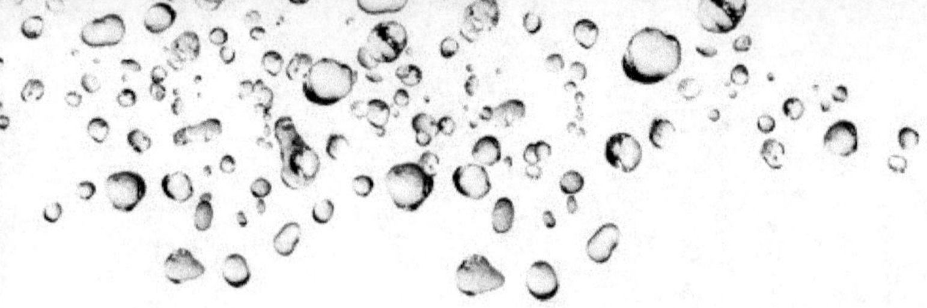

In order to maintain adequate hydration levels, please use the following guidelines

DRINK
3-4 LITRES PLAIN WATER A DAY

+ You may drink green tea on top of your daily water intake

+ If you need flavour, add lemon or lime

+ Limit diet drinks and artificial sweeteners

+ Do not drink high sugar or high calorie fruit juices

+ Black coffee is okay in moderation

+ Do not drink sports drinks for the sake of it, use only for training

+ Limit alcohol consumption to once a week as part of your cheat meal and a maximum of 3 glasses of wine

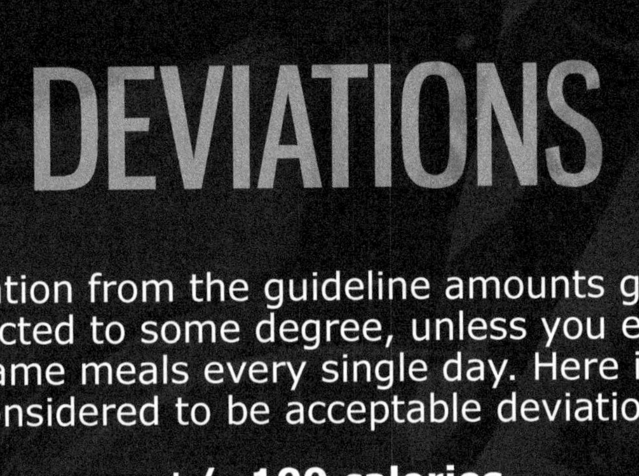

DEVIATIONS

Deviation from the guideline amounts given is expected to some degree, unless you eat the exact same meals every single day. Here is what is considered to be acceptable deviations:

+/- 100 calories

+/- 5g fat

+/- 10g carb

+/- 20g protein

Consistency is more important than perfection, however, if you are on the Trim phase and trying to lower your body fat levels, these deviations can cause plateaus. Therefore, if you do hit a sticking point try to rein this in and see if this kick starts your progress.

OVERVIEW

As you are probably aware, there are two basic types of cardio, low intensity and high intensity. The difference between the two types is based on how they are performed.

High intensity interval training (HIIT), is based on the principle of performing alternating periods of high and low intensity. An example of HIIT training is sprinting for 30 seconds, followed by 60 seconds rest and repeating for up to 30 minutes

Low intensity steady state cardio (LISS), on the other hand, is performed at a consistent and low to moderate intensity for the duration of the exercise. An example of LISS cardio is running or cycling for an hour. zzzzz

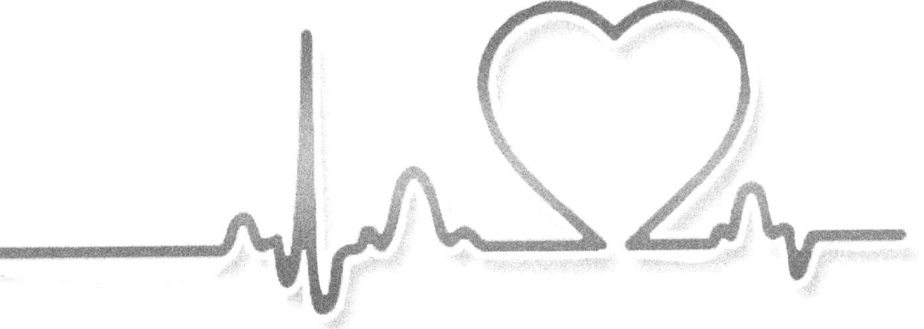

LEVELS

You'll want to work according to your level of fitness. As you get fitter, your breathing will become easier and recovery periods shorter. Therefore, you should regularly increase the level of intensity to to keep your body from acclimatising and slowing fat burning. Always keep the total time below 30 minutes, and adjust your intensity instead.

On the following pages are some examples of levels and progressions you can use, however, feel free to experiment and create a routine that works for you, these are only guidelines.

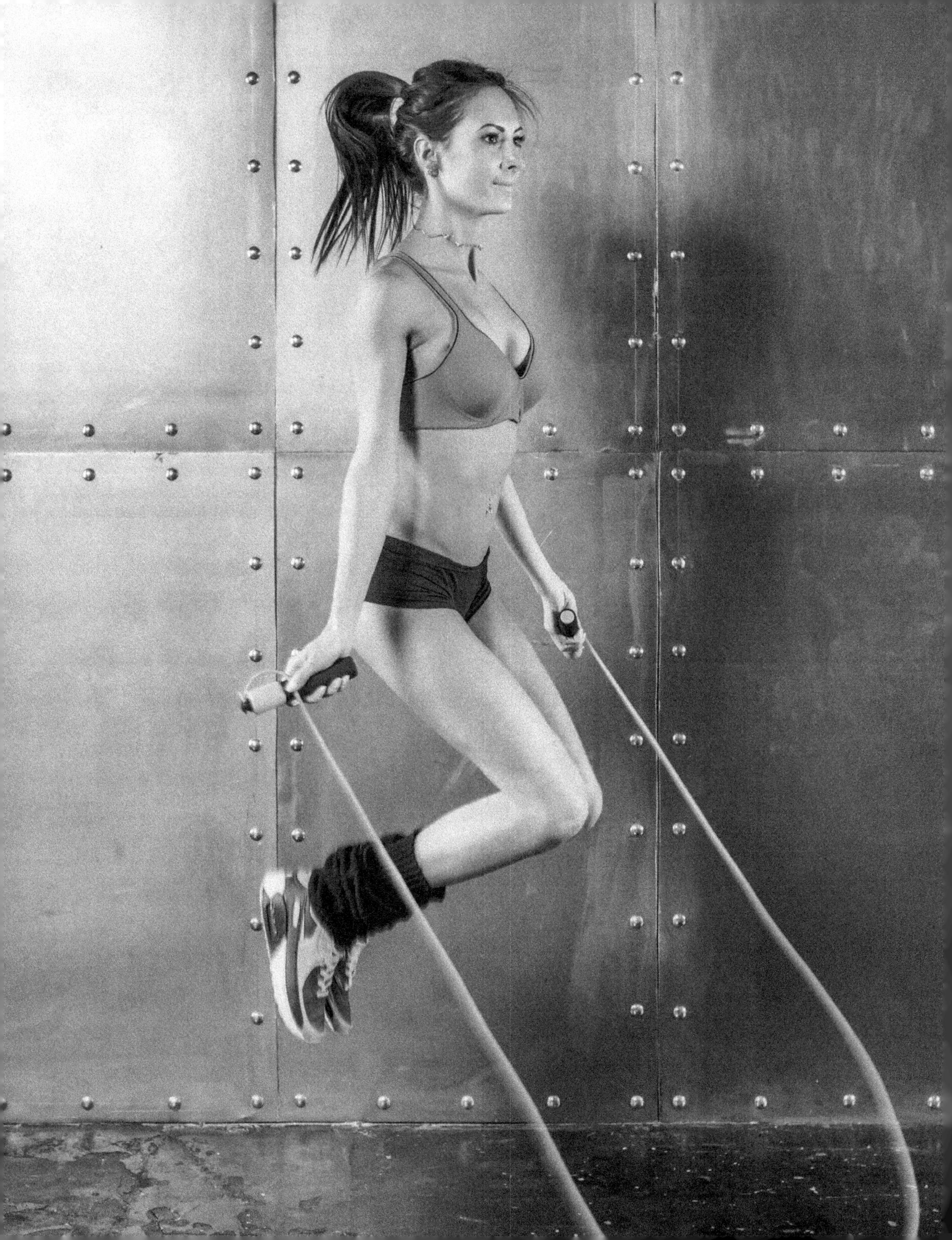

Now, don't get me wrong, there are fat burning and cardiovascular benefits associated with performing LISS cardio, however, as you're not looking to run a marathon as part of this program you really don't need lonnnnng cardio sessions slowing down your fat burning potential.

For the purposes of optimising body composition goals, HIIT training really is just far superior in every way. Here are the reasons why:

+ The after burn effect means you resting metabolic rate is increased for 24 hours after your session
+ Sessions are short, but so very effective
+ Improved insulin sensitivity means bye bye muffin top
+ Shorter sessions preserve your curves, aka muscles
+ Burns through a significant amount of body fat in much shorter periods
+ Increases your muscles' ability to burn fat for energy
+ Elevates growth hormone levels, which optimises fat loss and muscle growth
+ Releases chemicals that increase fat oxidation
+ Can reduce appetite

By far the greatest benefit of HIIT over LiISS is it's ability to preserve muscle while it burns huge amount of body fat. Longer sessions of cardio are proven to be more likely to burn muscle for fuel, which only serves to preserve the skinny fat cycle. That is not the look we are after.

Okay, so let's look at how to effectively incorporate HIIT protocols into your routine.

INTENSITY

The high intensity portions of your training should be to the point that you are breathing hard, approximately 90% effort. If you can talk while you're in the high intensity phase, you're not working hard enough and need to ramp up the intensity. You should also note that the high intensity intervals are supposed to be done fast and hard, not slow and hard. So only increase the resistance settings when your fitness has improved beyond your speed. Remember, sprinting, not jogging.

If you're using a machine for your intervals, it may take time for the machine to get up to speed so you'll want to start the speed increase a few seconds before your intensity is due to increase. You don't want to build up the effort, but rather launch into the high intensity portion immediately. Your breathing should become hard within 10-15 seconds thereafter.

The low intensity phases are active recovery periods, they are not rest periods. Therefore, you should keep moving at a steady pace during this low intensity phase. As a beginner, you'll want to start out with longer rest periods in the 1:2 ratio or more. As you get fitter, rest periods will reduce.

METHOD

HIIT cardio is typically performed biking, rowing or sprinting, however, it is not limited to those and can be performed using pretty much any type of exercise that can quickly increase and decrease intensity.

You could use jump ropes, elliptical, battle ropes and even plyometrics. You can perform them outdoors or indoors, with machines or without. The choice really is yours.

The only thing to note is that it is good to mix things up so that you're not using the same method all the time. The body is smart and will adapt over time, so get creative and have some fun experimenting.

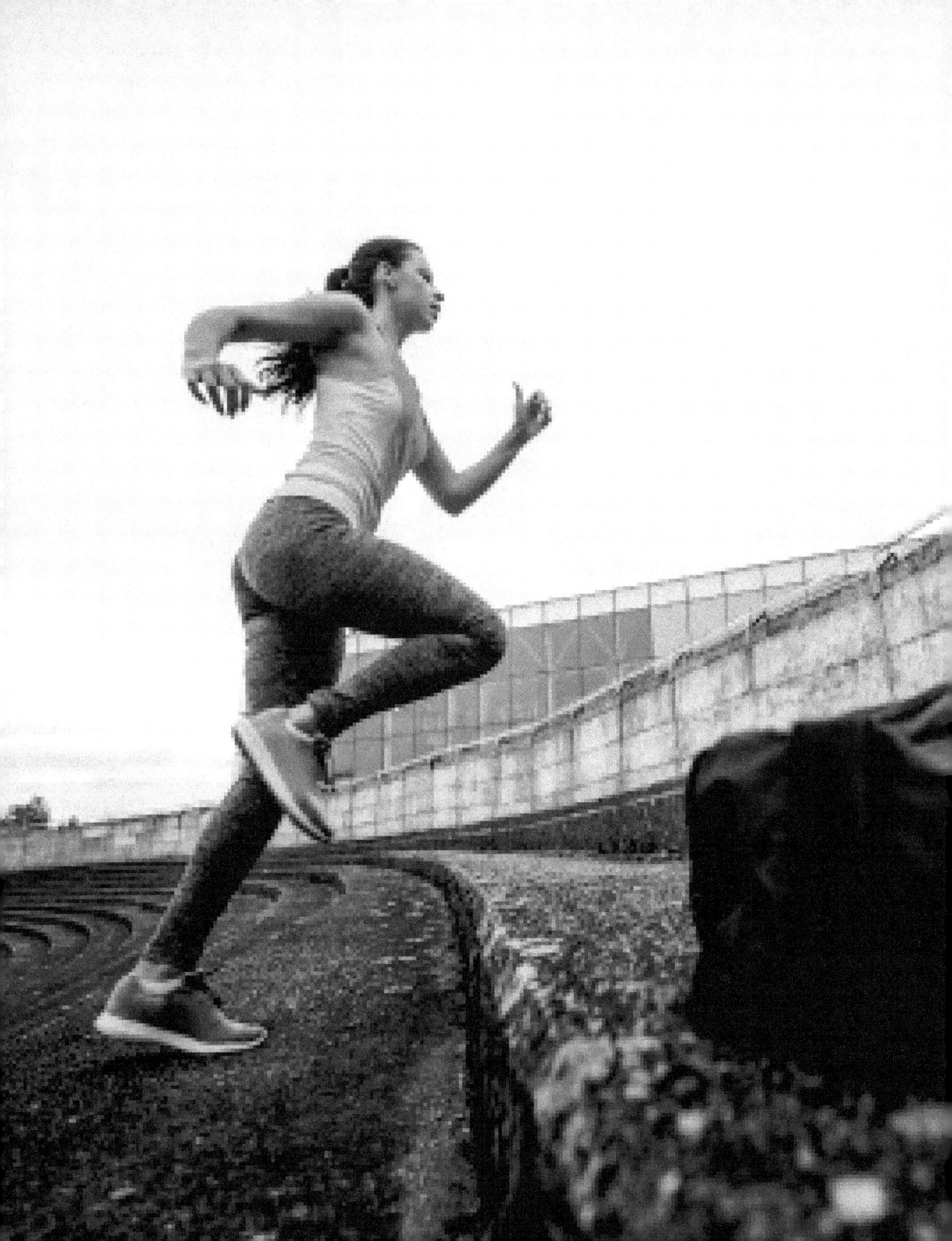

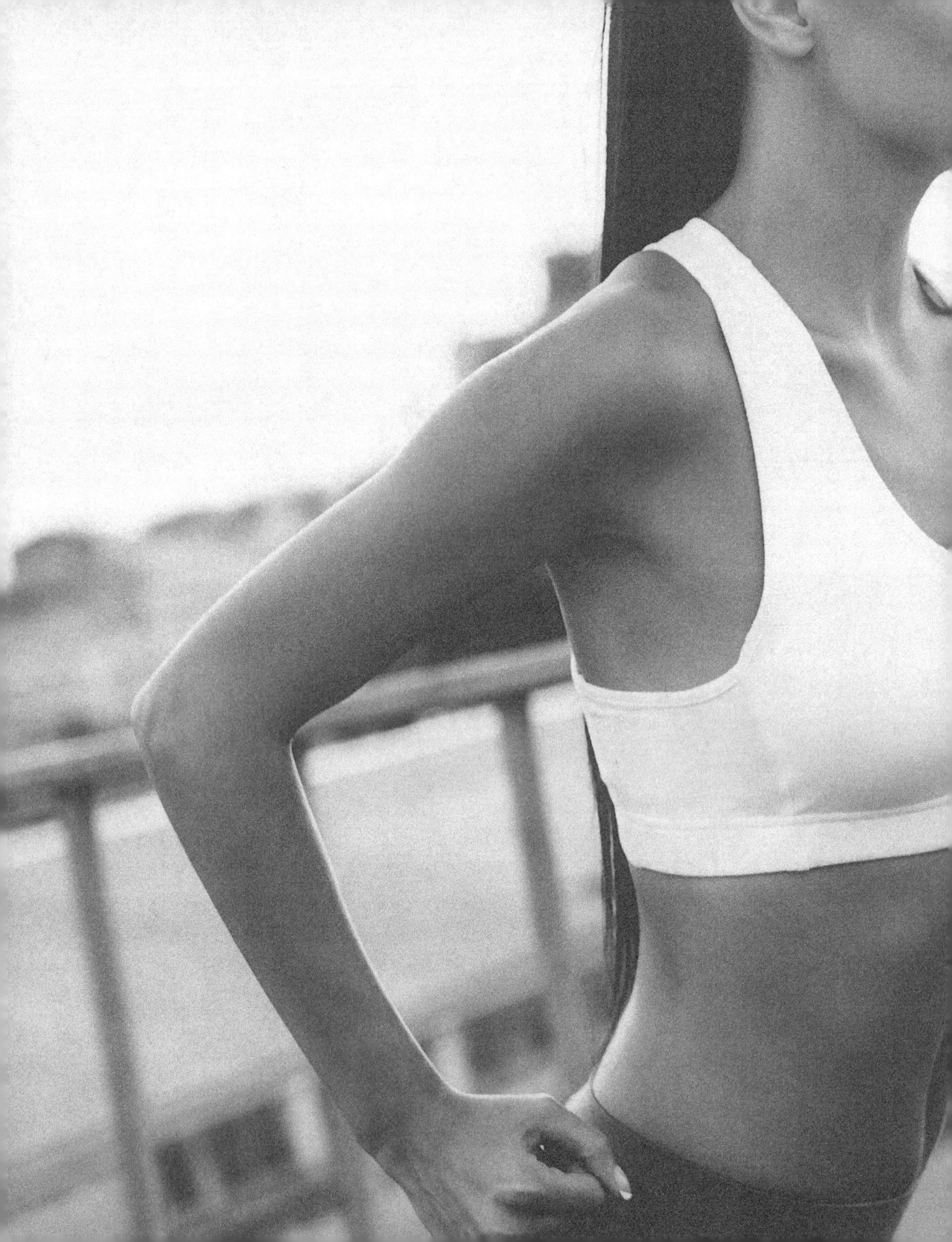

NO EQUIPMENT

BODY WEIGHT HIGH INTENSITY MOVES

Mountain climbers
Jumping lunges
High knees and kick butts
Jumping squats
Burpees
Frog jumps
Switch kicks
Jumping Jacks
Long jumps
Skater with touch down
Squat jumps
Shadow boxing
Sprinting
In and out jumps
Hill sprints

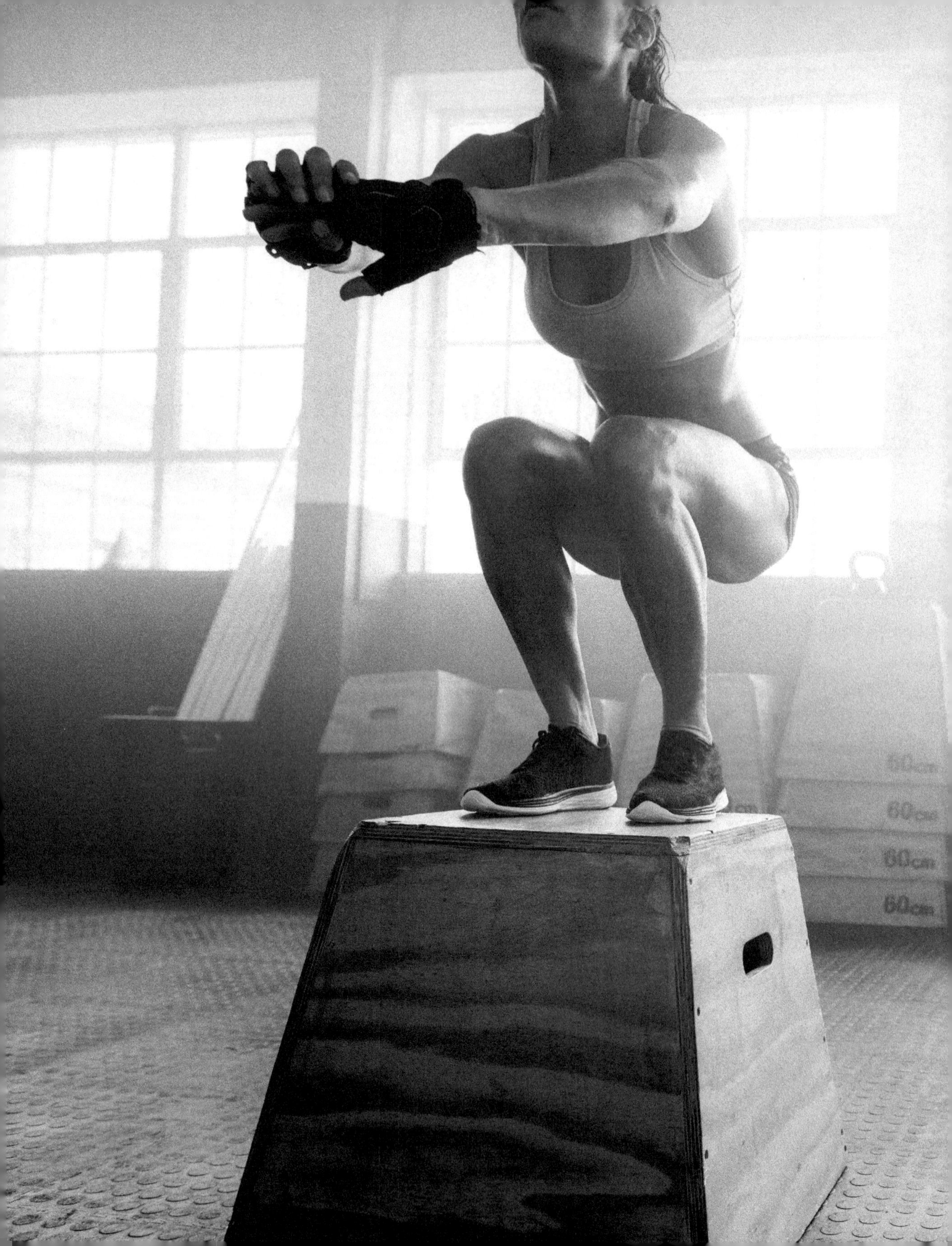
60cm
60cm
60cm
60cm

MINIMAL EQUIPMENT

HIGH INTENSITY MOVES

Box jumps
Punch bag boxing
Kettlebell swings
Skipping with rope
Boxing with friend
Battle ropes
Power skipping
Stair climbing

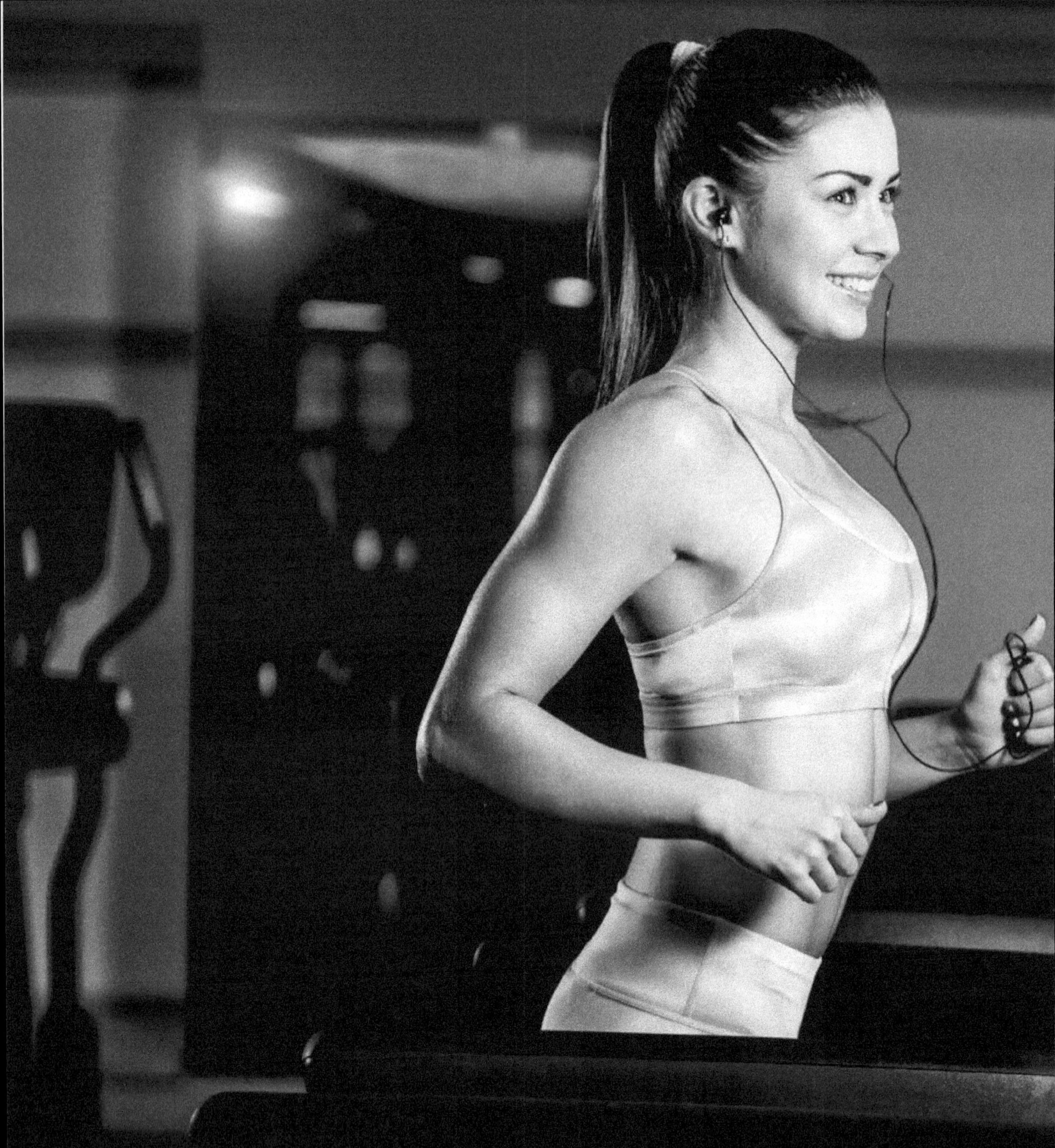

TREADMILL BASED

HIGH INTENSITY ADAPTATIONS

Forward frog jumps
Sideways jumping squats
Walking lunges
Elevated walking kick backs

CARDIO WITH WEIGHTS

As well as performing cardio the traditional way, you can also use weight training as a cardio tool. The benefit of weight based cardio is that the engagement of your muscles will amplify the afterburn effect, preserve your lean tissue and help build your definition all in once hit. It's an all round win-win.

There are several ways you can do weight based cardio, these are:

+ High rep with low rest periods
+ Alternate traditional cardio with weights
+ Plyometric based movements with weight of choice
+ Supersetting two exercises back to back with no rest
+ Combining two weight training moves into one fluid movement

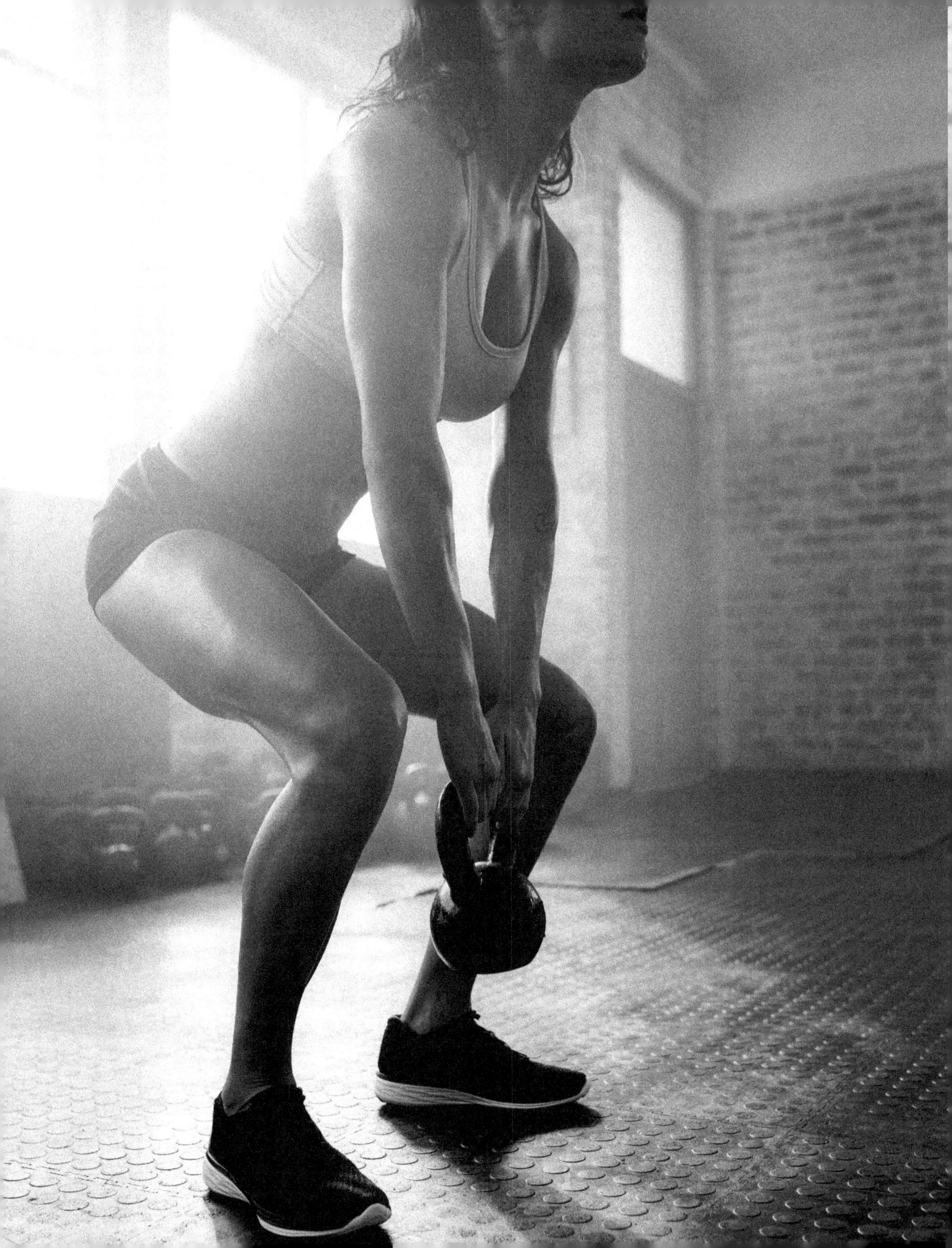

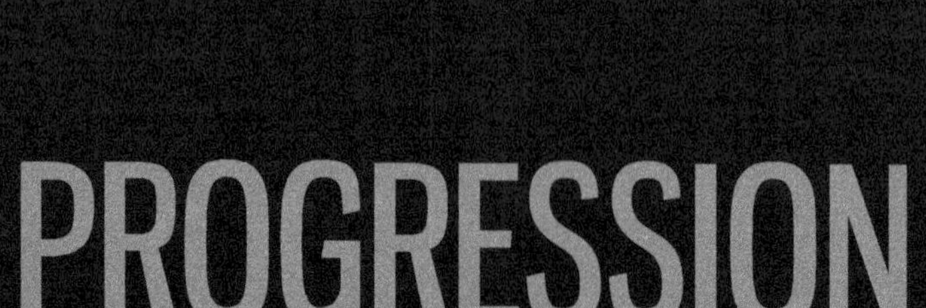

PROGRESSION

The body adapts to whatever loads you put it under so, Just like with training and nutritoin, you'll want to progressively adjust your cardio routine. This could be through intensity, duration, frequency or method.

Mix things up every two weeks or so and you'll see far greater results over time.

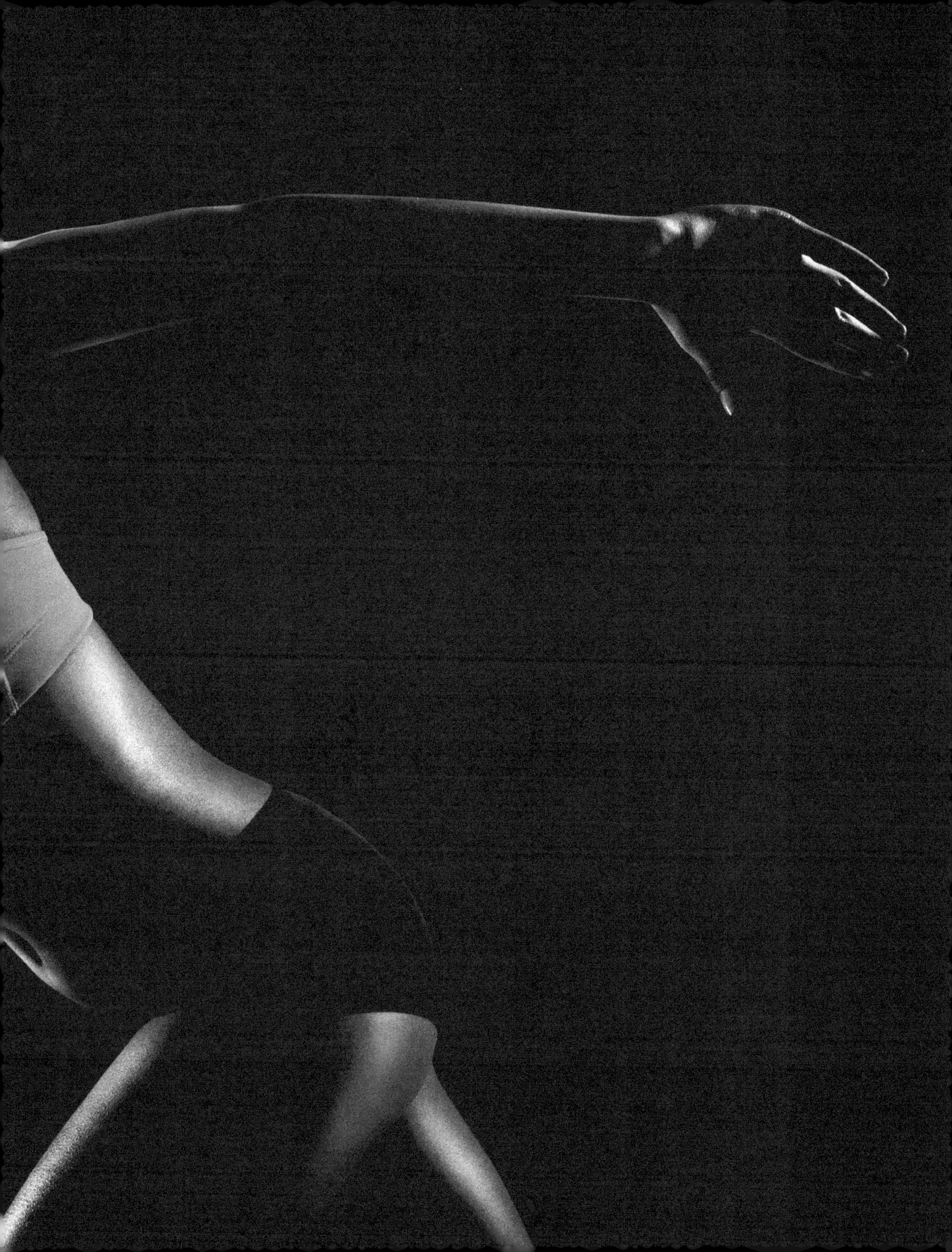

POST TRAINING
CARDIO

Aside from HIIT training, you may perform an additional 20-30 minutes LISS following your training session. After training, muscle glycogen is depleted and cardio during this period will act similar to that of performing fasted cardio. In other words, your body will turn immediately to fat stores for energy.

Be sure consume your post workout protein before this cardio to avoid muscle loss.

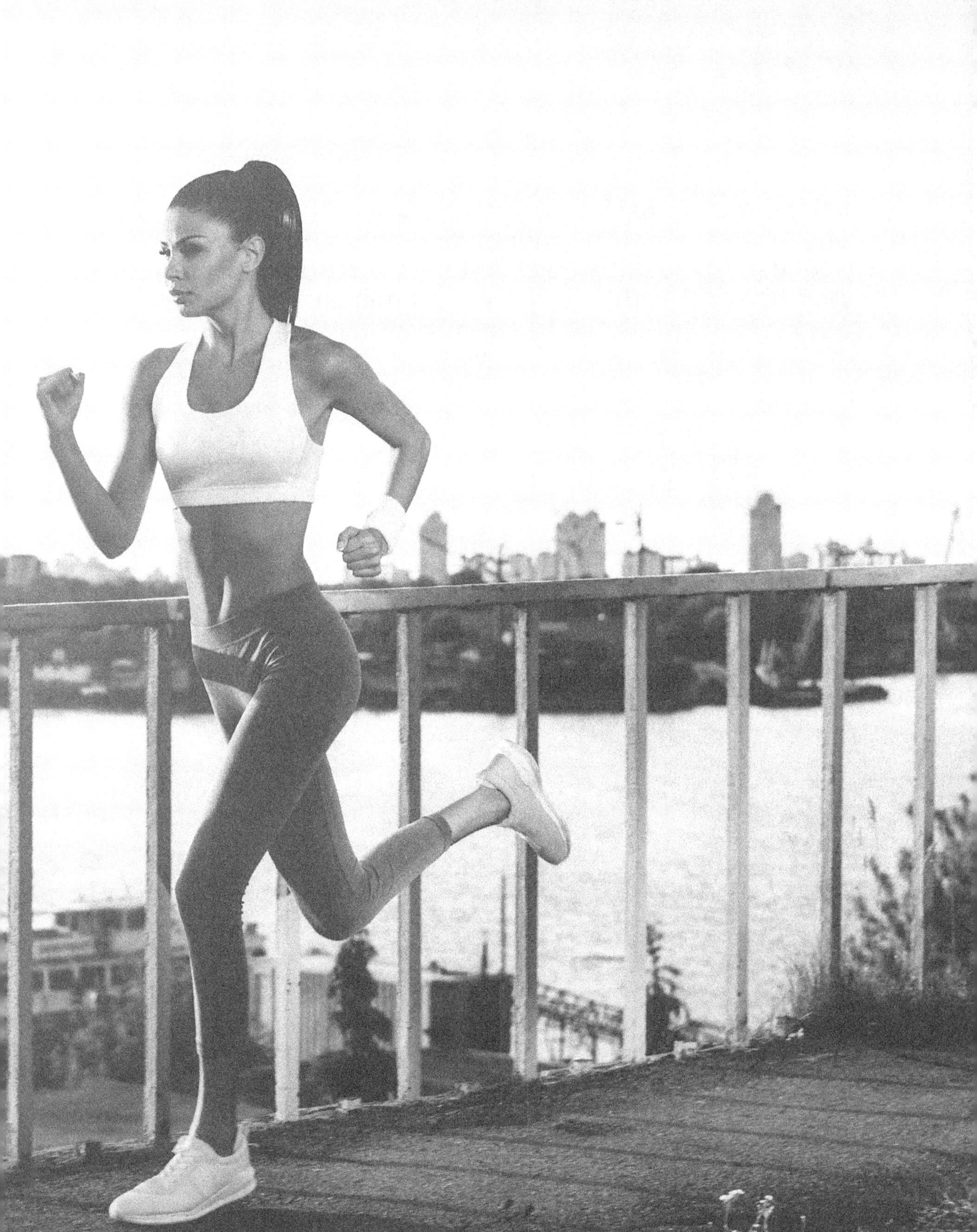

HOW IT WORKS

You'll be cycling back and forth between THE SCULPT PHASE and THE TRIM PHASE, depending on your how your body responds. The idea being to keep your metabolism firing and your body fat within lower, yet manageable levels, as you continue to carve your curves.

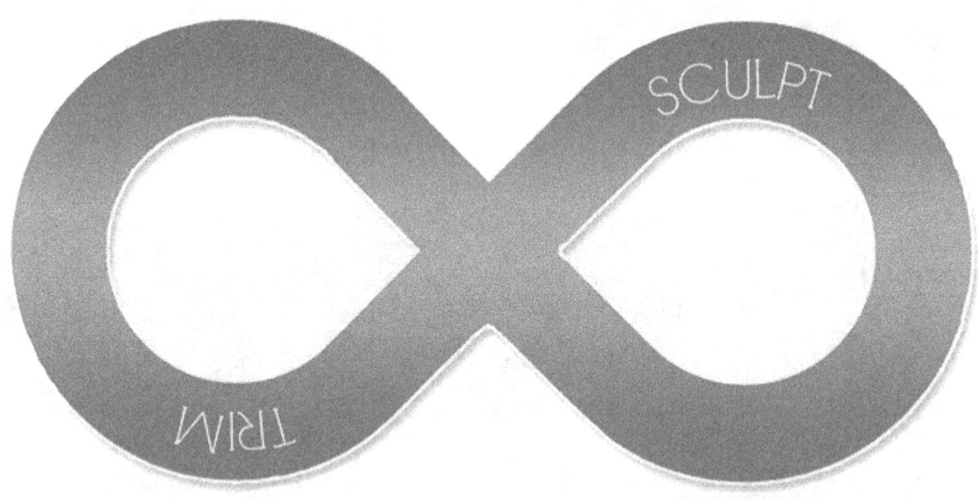

15-20% BODY FAT

Over the course of the program, you'll want to maintain a body fat percentage of between 15% and 20%.

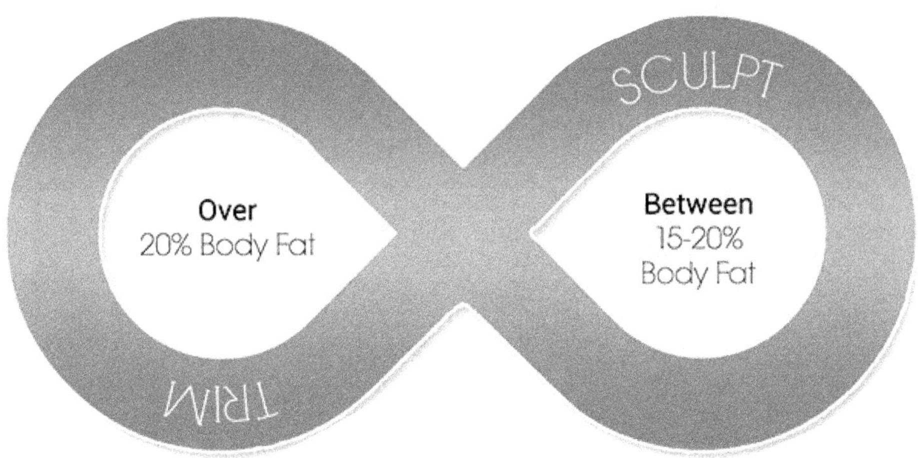

So, if your body fat levels are higher than 20% when starting the program, you'll begin on the trim phase so that you can bring those down to the 15-20% region. Once you get down to this level, or there about, you'll move onto the sculpt phase where you can really begin to sculpt and shape your curves. You'll want to remain on the sculpt phase throughout much of the program, only reverting back to the trim phase if your body fat increases above 20%.

BREAKING THE CYCLE

You can remain in the sculpt-trim loop for as long as you need. The only time you really need to break this cycle is when you are happy with your curves and want to enter ongoing maintenance which requires only 2 HIIT sessions a week..

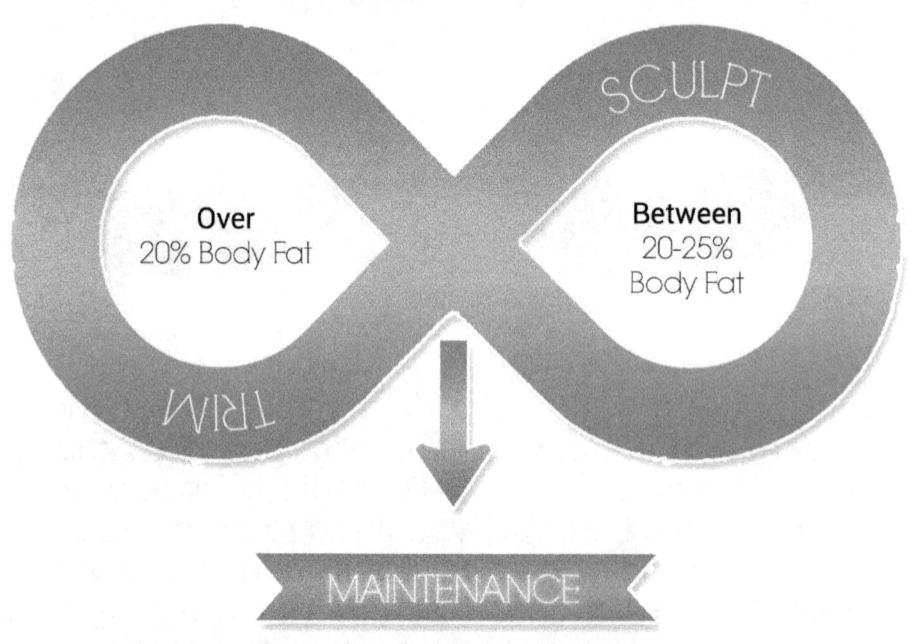

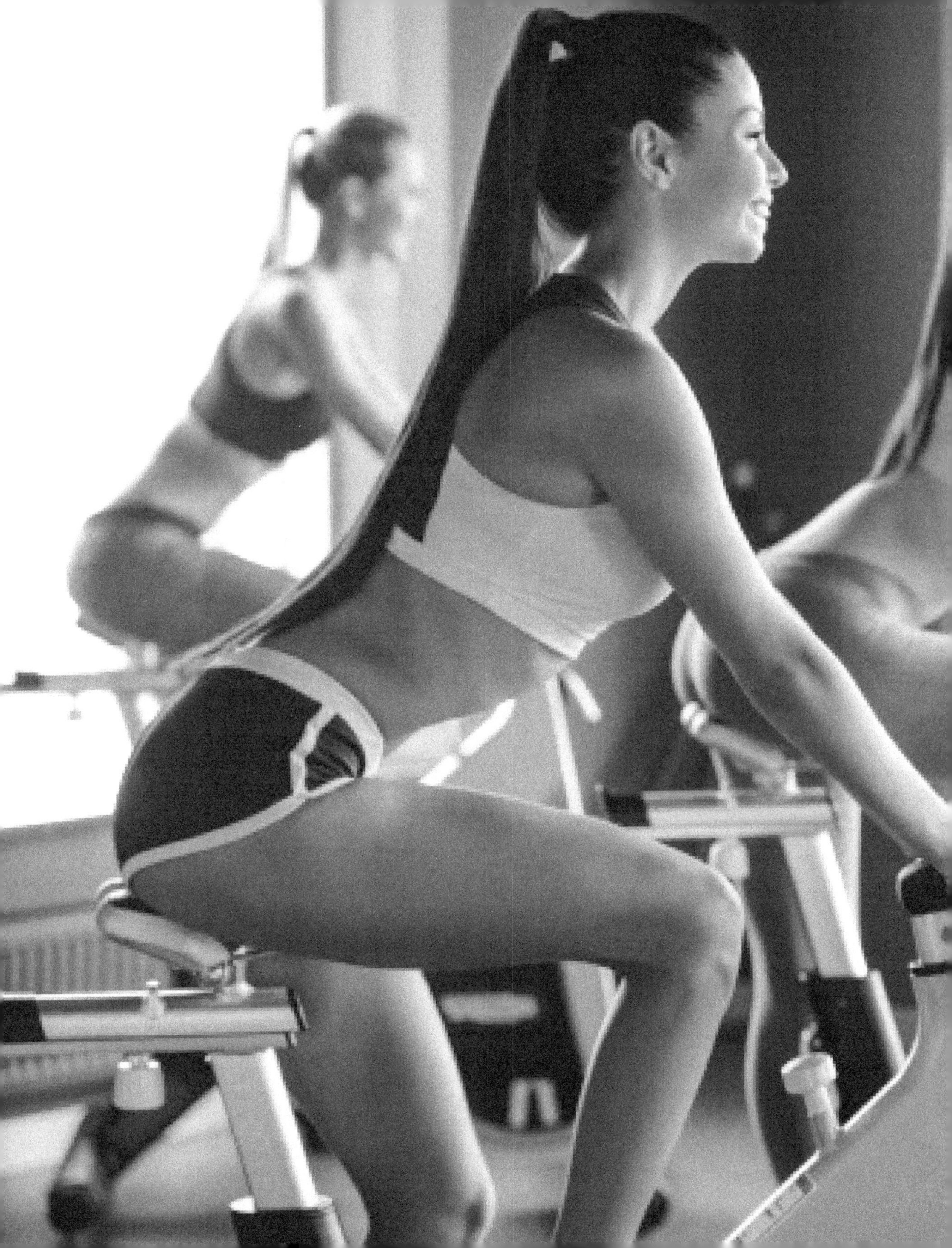

SCULPT PHASE

The goal within the Sculpt phase is to keep body fat levels under control, therefore, the frequency will remain consistent throughout the weeks totalling 60 minutes each week. Depending on your preference, level of fitness and schedule, we offer three choices of frequency and timing, these are:

4x 15 Minutes
3x 20 Minutes
2x 30 Minutes

Of course, you may rotate these to add more variety too.

TROUBLESHOOTING

FAT LOSS PROGRESS

If you have found your fat loss progress stalling, take a look at the list below and be honest with yourself.

TRAINING

- Are you training hard enough?
- Are your HIIT intervals intensive enough?
- Are you giving 100% in all areas?
- Are you skipping cardio or adding extra cardio?
- Are you missing training seasons or cutting them short?

DIET

- Are you following the guidelines?
- Are you adding extras? Not weighing food, adding oils and sugary sauces
- Are you eating in restaurants too often? restaurants will add more oils and sugars than you expect and calories add up unknowingly
- Are you having too much salt?
- Are you having too many cheats or too much food for your off plan meal?
- Are you doing refeeds, have you read and understand the guidance?
- Are you macro tracking if so are you over or under eating? Make sure you include supplements and ensure food nutrition is input correctly into the tracking software (create custom foods on the software to ensure accuracy if necessary)
- Are you spacing your meals out during the day
- Are you measuring correctly? Weighing cooked meats?

FLUIDS

- Are you drinking enough water? 3-6 litres daily?
- Are you drinking alcohol?
- Are you drinking calories in fruit juices and fizzy drinks or milk in tea and coffee
- Are you using diuretics, herbal diuretics or teas? These will make you lighter one day but you might find you get a water rebound the next day. Steer clear, its not good for the body to be constantly dehydrated

GENERAL

- Have you read all the documents in the program? You might be missing some vital information

In the case that you are doing everything correctly and still not seeing results you can look at adjusting your calorie deficit, or reducing your carbs a little further. If you have a serious problem with fat loss and are genuinely giving your best, I recommend going to your doctor and asking for a thyroid and hormone profile blood test.

FREQUENTLY

ASKED QUESTIONS

Q: I've eaten something that wasn't on the plan, what should I do?

Sometimes cravings and temptations get the better of you. Don't allow this to take you off track or dampen your drive. Consistency is better than perfection and slight deviations here and there are to be expected. Life happens. As long as you're hitting your program 90% of the time, these little hiccups can be offset most of the time.

There are a few ways to deal with this scenario. You could redistribute your remaining calories for the rest of the day to compensate, you'll be surprised what reducing your meals by just 25-50 calories can do to rein in those calories. Or, if you feel the food will have severely impacted your progress, you can use that as your cheat meal and forego your scheduled cheat meal. Whatever you do, don't amp up your cardio or you'll burn out.

Q: I am so sore, I don't think I can manage another workout. What can I do?

Soreness in the early stages can be quite severe, and you'll not want to be training while they are in their most severe stages because that's when your muscles need recovery time. You'll experience this quite a lot in the first few weeks while your body becomes accustomed to the training, so take heed, it will reduce.

There are several remedies that may help reduce the soreness. You can take a hot bath, take a walk, perform some light stretching, have a soft tissue massage, go for a swim and rest. If you find your muscles are still sore when you come to train that body part again, select an alternative day training session and come back to that muscle when it's recovered.

Q: I'm struggling with the HIIT's

HIIT training is supposed to be difficult and in the early days when you are building your stamina, it'll take some time to get used to it. Just take baby steps and do the very best you can. Start out with two separate sessions if you find that helps and just keep getting better.

Q: I feel uncomfortable in the gym, what shall I do?

It is easy to feel intimidated when you first enter the gym, particularly the free weights area where all the big beefy guys hang out. I felt this way too when I first joined. You'll actually find that most guys are more concerned with checking themselves out in the mirror than they are of you, and others are more than happy to assist if you ask. So, go in there and just do your thing. You'll soon feel right at home.

If you're still unsure, go ask one of the members of staff to show you how to use the equipment. This will help ease you into he environment without too much attention, and you'll have the added benefit of being show how to use everything without having to work it out for yourself. In fact, as a beginner to weights, I'd highly recommend this approach anyway. If you can afford one, you could also enlist the help of a personal trainer to take you through a few sessions until you find your confidence.

Q: The scale weight has increased. I'm freaking out

As we covered in the body composition guide, putting on weight is not a problem and scale weight is irrelevant. Get off that horrible contraption and go re-read the body composition guide to refresh your memory on wha tis important. As long as you've been doing the weight training sessions and sticking to healthy nutrition as per the program outline, the weight is more than likely muscle and/or water weight. If I forgot to say it before, leave those scales alone lady.

Q: I feel hungry all the time, what should I do?

When you're in a caloric deficit, hunger is just part of the game. However, if your hunger is quite severe, recalculate your calorie intake and adjust if it needs updating. Next, check your water intake is between 3-4 litres a day as thirst can feel like hunger. If both of these are correct, you could try increasing your vegetable intake or add an additional protein shake before your training. If after doing all the above you are still ravenous, you could try reducing your calorie deficit. You've been provided with two ranges, 15-20% and 20-25%, so give the lower deficit range a go and see how you feel.

Q: There's so much food, do I have to eat it all?

Because the foods on this program are highly nutritious, the volume of food can appear to be high. The same may be true if you have been on highly restrictive calorie diets or usually eat a lot of fast food that has more calories, but is not nutritious. If you struggle to fit the meals in, you can break them down into smaller portions which will make it more manageable. Or you could substitute some of the whole foods with lighter equivalents, such as swapping out a chicken breast for a protein shake. .

Q: I'm struggling to find time and keep missing meals

Preparation is the key to success. If time is an issue, prepare a batch of meals all at once so you have less cooking to do. Distribute those into containers and you have your meals at the ready. No excuses.

Q: The training is beyond my ability, what can I do?

Do as much as you can. Something is better than nothing, and as long as you keep putting in the effort, the changes will come. If your form is a problem, seek assistance from a member of the gym staff, a personal trainer or a movement specialist. It's expected during the early stages that you'll find things a challenge. It shows you're doing something beyond your comfort zone, and that's where the changes take place. Keep going and you'll soon get stronger. .

Q: Can I do yoga on my off days?

Yes, yoga is a great addition to the training program and is highly encouraged to retain your flexibility.

Q: I've never worked out before and the first workout KICKED MY BUTT. What should I do?

First, kudos to you for starting! Challenge is a good thing-injury is not. You should expect to be out of breath, to be mentally pushed to finish the workout, and to be a little sore the following day-but you should not feel unsafe or beyond your capabilities. So make sure to modify the moves as mentioned in the descriptions and go at your own pace. If it says 3 sets and you can only do 2 that is fine. Do 3 the next week and progress at a speed that is right for you. Just keep trying your best and your abilities will increase.

Q: Can I do more exercises for my abs?

The prescribed amount of ab exercises have been kept to a minimum to create a particular outcome, however, this program is and how you use it is your choice. If you like the look of more defined abs, by all means increase those exercises. I'd still recommend avoiding oblique training however as this will bulk your curves too much. .

Q: What if I just jump right into the advanced program even though I'm not ready for it?

Go about things wisely and start at the bottom and move up gradually. There's no rush and you'll progress much faster if you start with a level you are ready for. Continual progression is the key to changes, not using all your tools at once and burning out.

THE S.T.E.P FORMULA

The female fitness formula to perfect proportions

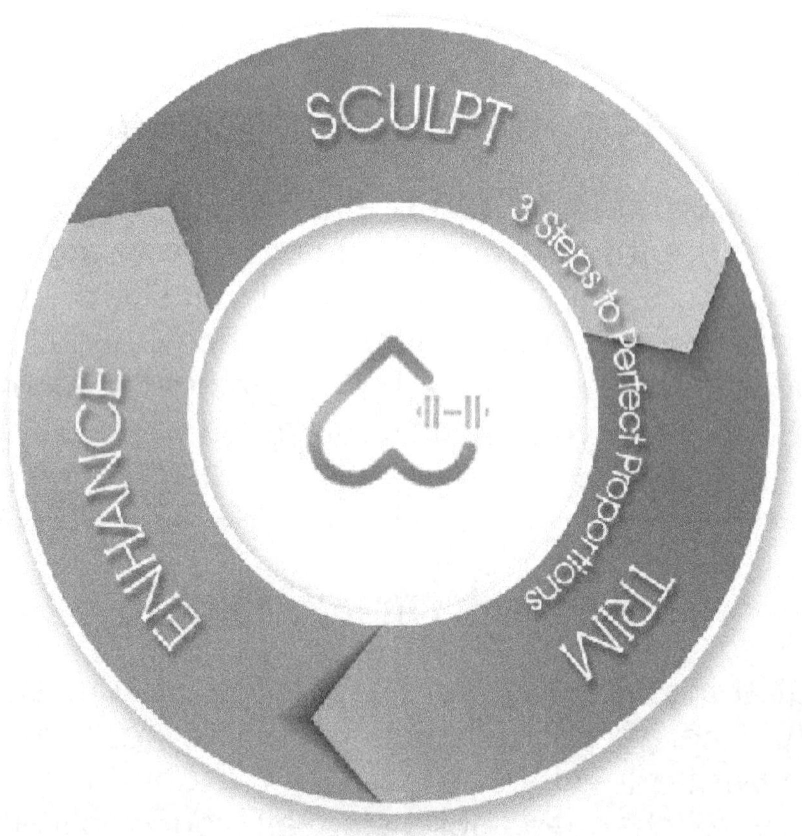

SCULPT + TRIM + ENHANCE = PERFECT PROPORTIONS

The S.T.E.P Formula™ incorporates a specialised combination of cardiovascular and weight training guidelines, alongside a balanced and healthy nutrition plan and 100% healthy supplements.

Each phase of the S.T.E.P Formula™ is distinct and unique in it's own right, however, each phase works in tandem to get you results in the most efficient way possible. This means there is no need to wait until you hit the latter phase for changes to to be seen, because we will show you how to make the most of your curves from day one.

Let's take a brief look through the main focus areas of each phase so you know what you can expect as you embark on your journey to your perfect DreamGirl™ proportions.

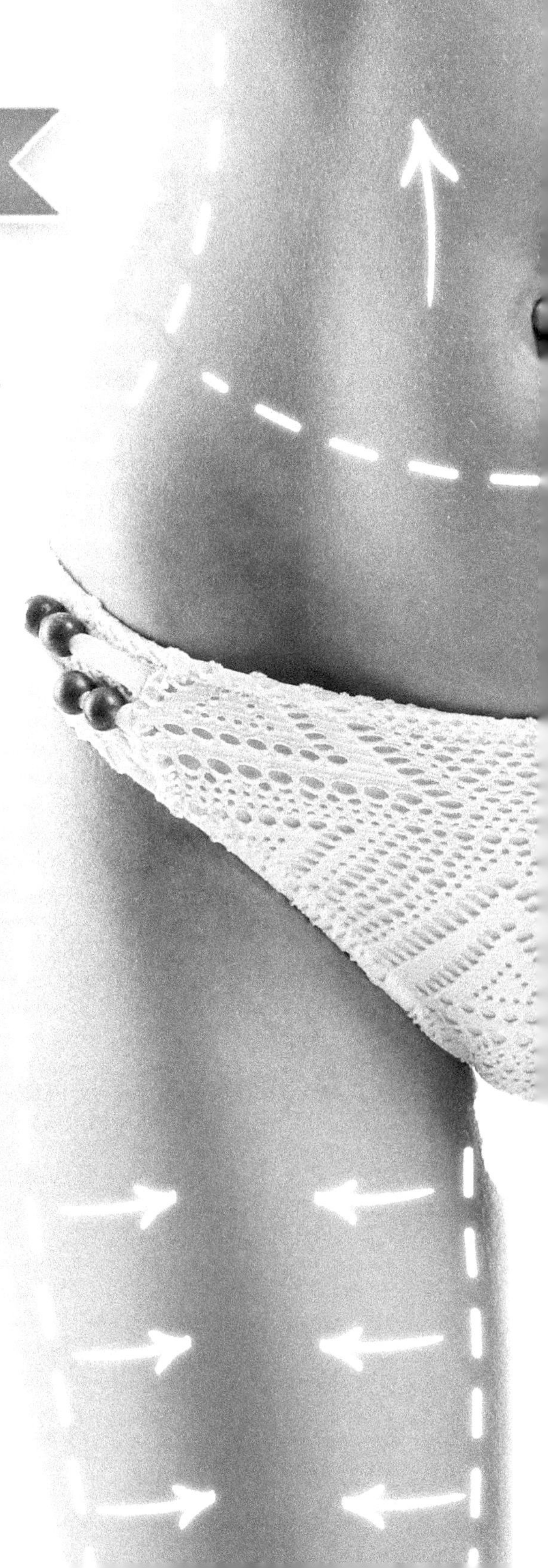

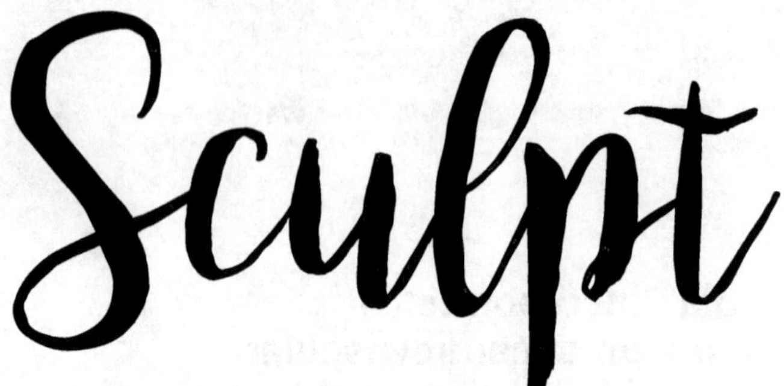

The sculpt phase is the most critical of all three phases. The focus of the sculpt phase is two-fold:

SCULPT YOUR CURVES

To sculpt out the curves of your body, we'll use carefully selected targeted training techniques.

TRANSFORM YOUR BODY COMPOSITION

Body composition is vital to transforming your body from soft and shapeless from tight and toned,

The training I will introduce you to is designed to sculpt the coveted and sexy hourglass shape, in a way that achieves balance and symmetry that is in accordance with your individual body shape.

You'll also learn how to avoid all the common mistakes and pitfalls associated with training incorrectly.

As your body composition changes within this phase, you'll notice an increase in lean body mass, and this is what will give you the firm and toned appearance you are looking to achieve.

There are two critical elements we will look at that will help you achieve your perfect DreamGirl™ proportions, these are:

INTRODUCE THE RIGHT TRAINING

AVOID THE WRONG TRAINING

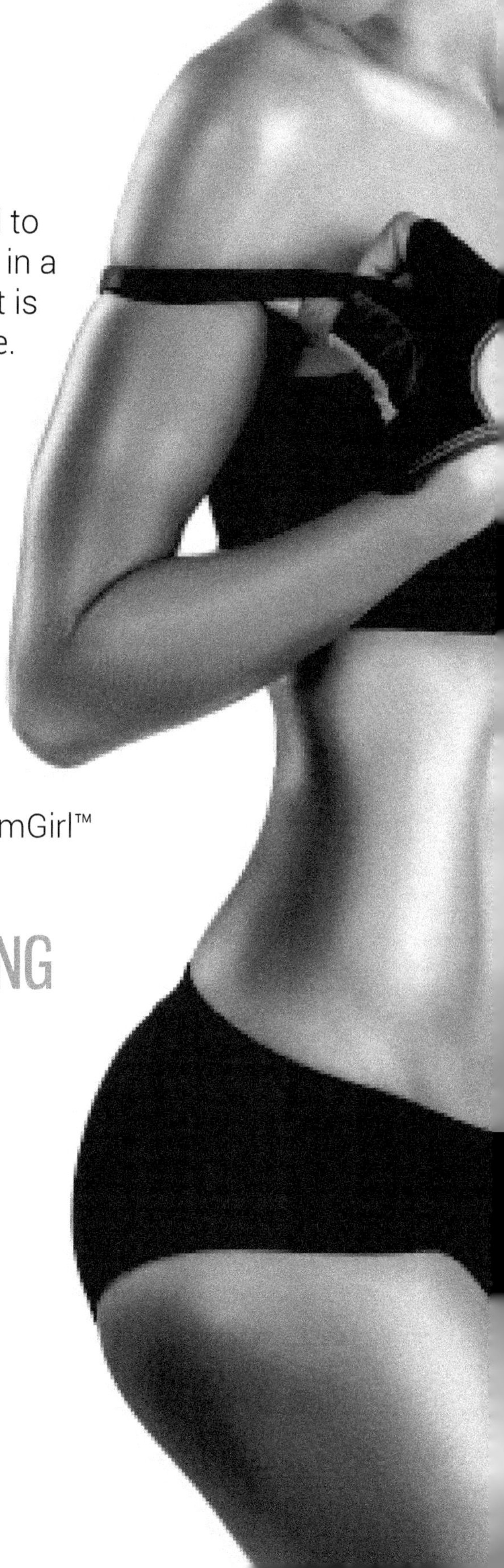

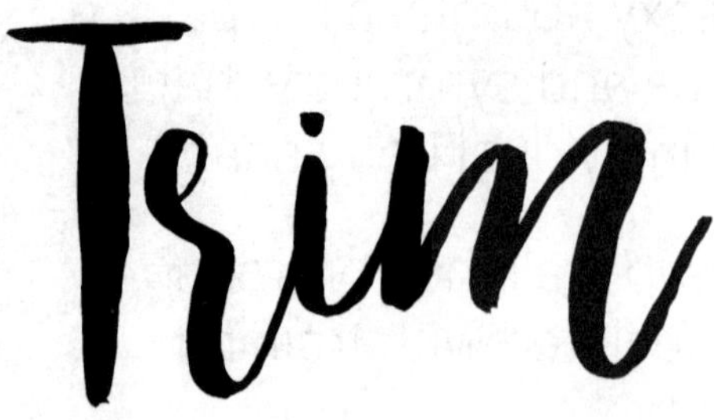

A tight and toned body doesn't come from training alone, it comes from reducing your body fat levels, and in the trim phase, we will torch your body fat to reveal your sexy womanly curves.

The trim phase is made up of two distinct elements:

INTRODUCE EFFECTIVE CARDIO SESSIONS

No long boring sessions

EAT FOODS THAT SUPPORT YOUR GOALS

Nope, not chicken and brocolli or rabbit food

Enhance

DreamCurves™ is a complete system, and the program wouldn't be complete without showing you how to further enhance your results. You'll discover:

WHAT SUPPLEMENTS SUPPORT YOUR GOALS

No crazy pill popping and no endorsements

HOW TO ELIMINATE LOVE HANDLES AND MUFFIN TOPS CAUSED BY HORMONE IMBALANCES

Hormones play such a huge role in body composition and how our bodies store fat, you may be surprised by what you discover here.

HOW IT WORKS

Each phase works in unison and you'll be cycling back and forth between the sculpt and the trim phase, depending on your how your body responds. The idea is to keep your metabolism firing and your body fat within lower, yet manageable levels, as you continue to carve your curves.

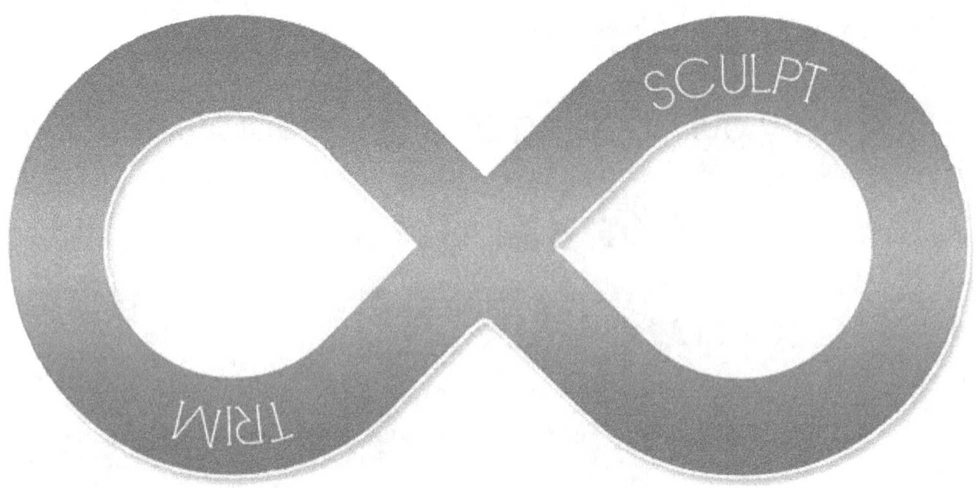

You'll want to maintain a body fat percentage of between 15% and 20%.

WHAT BODY FAT LEVEL?

The ideal level of body fat you can expect to achieve on this program is one whereby you have some visible muscular definition and are able to maintain a toned look year round, but not so much that your health and wellbeing is compromised or you begin to lose shape.

For this purpose, you'll be looking to achieve a lean, but healthy, body fat level of between 15-20%, depending on your preferences and how your body responds.

Going lower than this is possible, but that's going into the realms of advanced show prep and is not included as part of this program.

Be sure to sign up to the DreamGirl newsletter however as I'm going to be releasing a prep program in the near future.

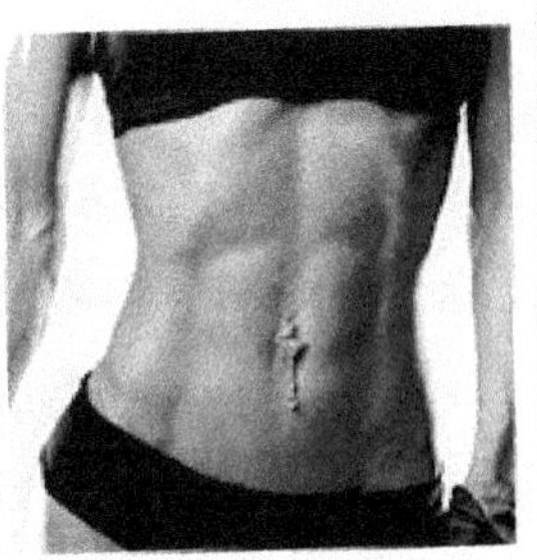

10-12%

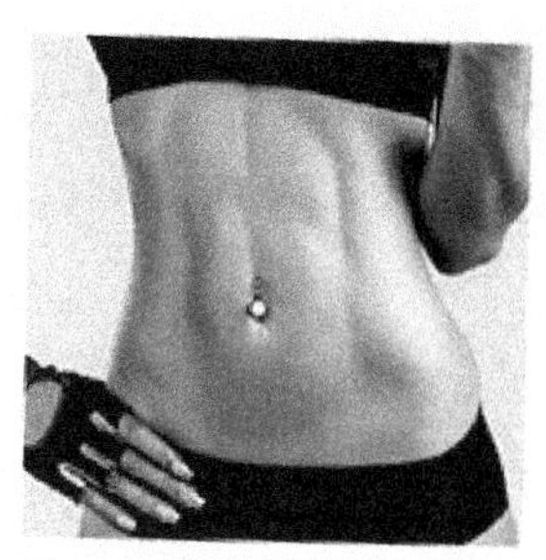

15-17%

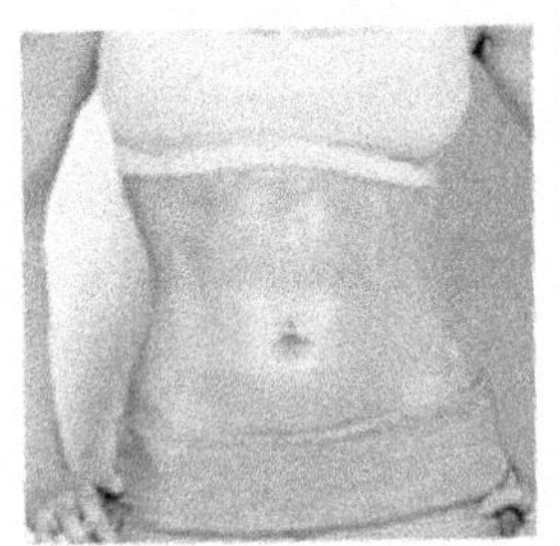

18-20%

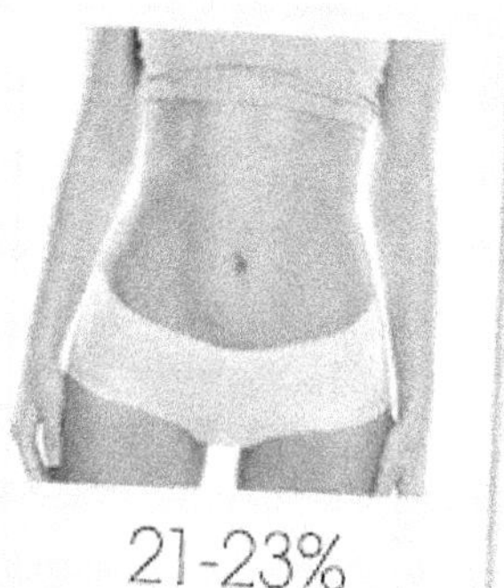

21-23%

So, if your body fat levels are higher than 20% when starting the program, you'll begin on the trim phase so that you can bring those down to the 15-20% region.

Once you get down to this level, you'll move onto the sculpt phase where you can really begin to sculpt and shape your curves.

The sculpt phase is ongoing because that's where you'll be shaping your body, and you'll only need to revert back to the trim phase if your body fat increases above 20%.

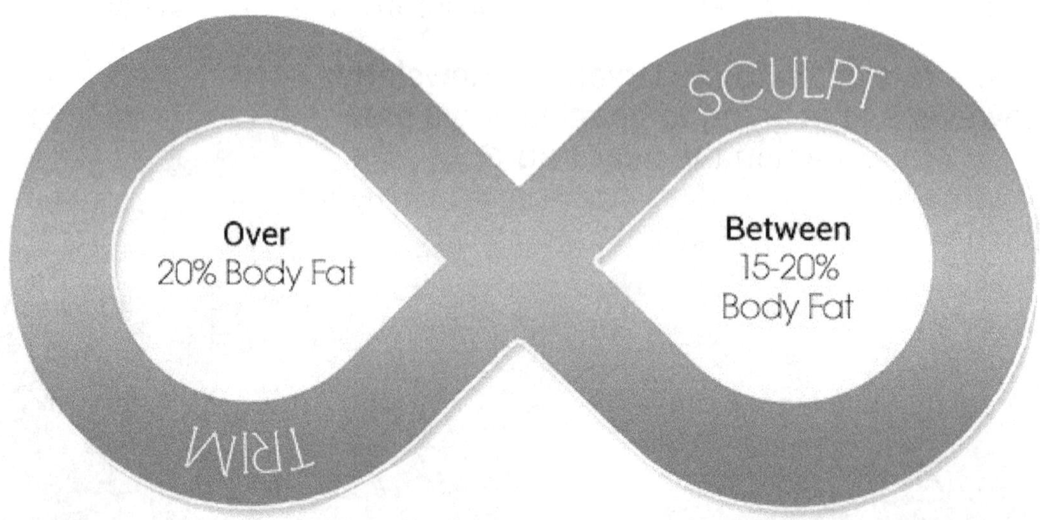

BREAKING THE CYCLE

You can remain in the sculpt-trim loop for as long as you need. The only time you really need to break this cycle is when you are happy with your curves and want to enter ongoing maintenance.

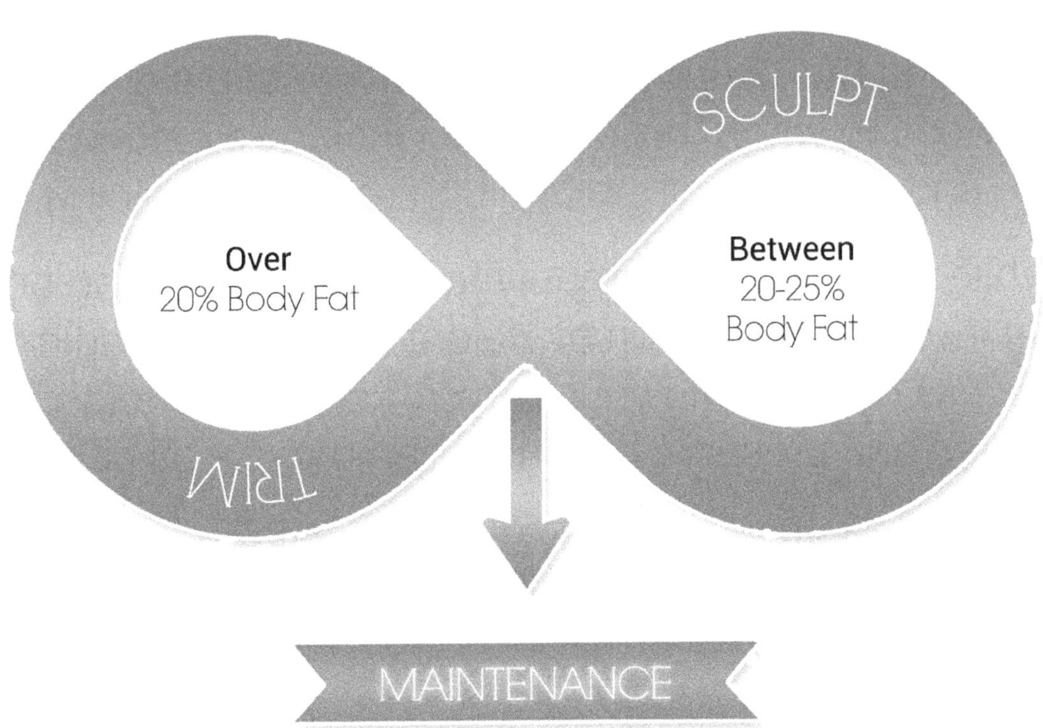

THE TRIM PHASE IS IDEAL IF:

+ Your body fat is above 20%
+ You haven't just come out of an extreme diet
+ You're an endomorph body type

If you have excess body fat, we first need to bring it down to around the 15-20% mark so that we can see what we are working with. This phase will include a caloric deficit and some cardio, in addition to weight training.

While this phase is primarily focused on reducing body fat levels, the addition of weight training will begin the process of sculpting your curves, keep your metabolism revved and preserve as much lean muscle as possible.

If you are already relatively lean, you may skip this stage and progress straight to the sculpt phase.

THE SCULPT PHASE IS IDEAL IF:

+ Your body fat is below 20%
+ You're an ectomorph body type

The sculpt phase is designed for those who have lower levels of body fat around the 15-20% mark.

During this phase, you'll increase calories and decrease cardio, focusing more on sculpting your curves, and increasing overall body composition.

You'll begin to see increased muscle tone, sexy curves and balance in your proportions during this stage.

Not sure what body type you are?
Don't worry, I'll cover this in a later section

TO ACHIEVE MAXIMUM RESULTS

While each of these phases are distinct and unique in their own right, you'll notice that each overlaps one another also. So, even in the Trim phase, there will be Sculpt phases elements, and vica versa.

The reason for this is to ensure your body composition benefits from an all round approach.

For example:

While in the Sculpt phase, Trim phase elements such as HIIT training and calorie cycling are still included, thereby avoiding any uneccessary weight gain while still developing your curves to a high degree.

Likewise, in the Trim phase you'll also find Sculpt phase body sculpting resistance training and this will enable you to drop body fat and keep your metabolism high, without compromising your lean body tissue.

And that is just how simple the steps are. So, now that you understand the basic steps, it's time to look at how to introduce them into your lifestyle so that you can achieve the results you want.

LET'S *transform* YOUR BODY...

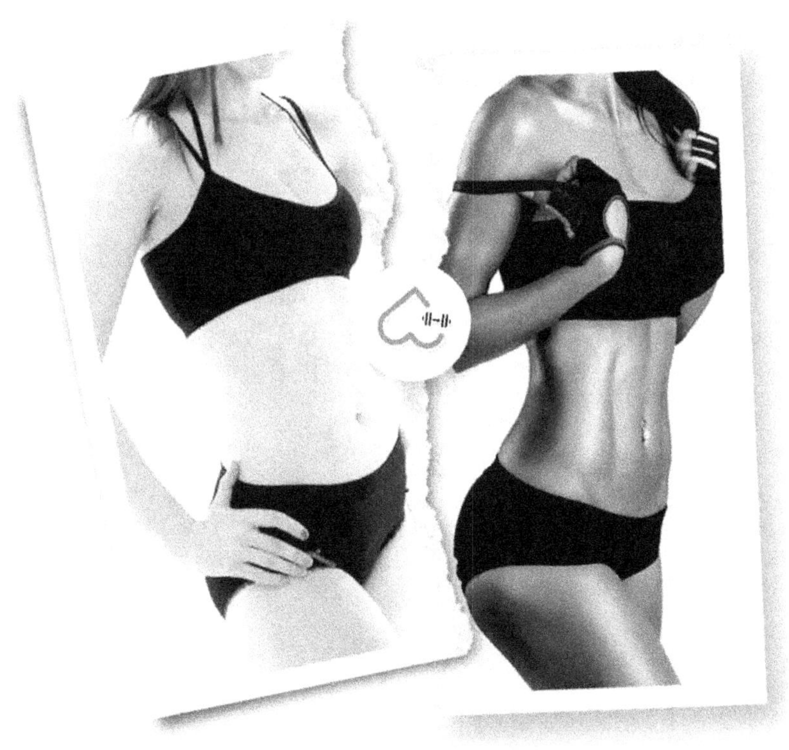

STEP ONE
READ THROUGH THE INFORMATION

This program is fairly thorough because I wanted you to fully understand why the program has been set out the way it has. So many fitness programs give a plan without the information to back it up, and I didn't want to do that because I think you deserve to understand the ideas backing it. I also wanted you to gain a better understanding of fat loss and body composition in general, so you can understand how things work for yourself. You shouldn't have to rely on expensive trainers for the rest of your life, and now you don't have to.

I suggest taking a relaxing evening to look through and digest the information before starting to put it to use. You'll be in a much better position to take action once you have the cognitive understanding.

STEP TWO
GO SHOPPING

You're going to need to stock up on some essentials before you officially begin. So take a look through the supplementation, grocery and equipment list to find out what you need, and then go grab those items.

You'll find the details for these in the following guidebooks:

+ Supplementation Guidelines
+ Nutrition Guidelines
+ Training Companion Guide

STEP THREE
GET MEASURING

Before you can start, you need to find out where you're starting from.

Take a look through the **Success Tracking Guidebook** and then begin to fill out the corresponding sections in your

Dream Journal.

This is the most exciting bit, because you'll not remain in the same condition for long. Say goodbye to your former self, and say hello to your future DreamGirl. Woo hoo.

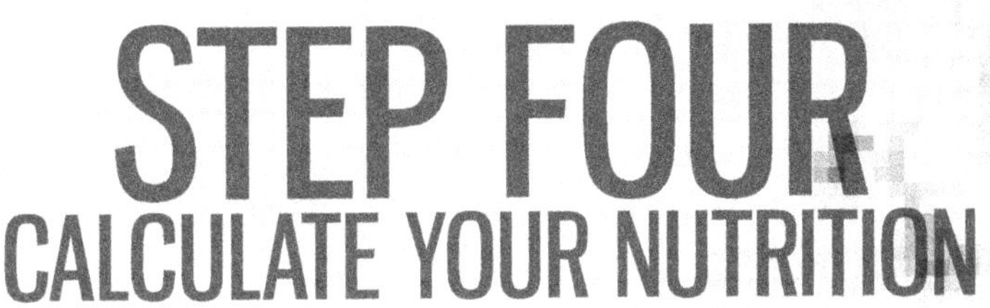

STEP FOUR
CALCULATE YOUR NUTRITION

With your measurements to hand, skip ahead to the **Nutrition Guidelines** so you can determine your caloric and macronutrient requirements.

GIVE YOURSELF

CHANCE TO SUCCEED

The idea of this program is to help you build new habits. This is not a short term get skinny hardcore diet program, it is a body composition program and I want you to learn to follow and stick to a healthy and focused routine that is sustainable for the rest of your life. No more fad diets, rebounding weight gain or skinny fat syndrome. This program is manageable, it is sustainable, and it is effective.

Having said that, the starting point is always the hardest because you'll be building new habits and will want to see results overnight. You will see results, but you'll need to remain compliant to see them. Don't worry though, I've factored in plenty of rest and some satisfyingly awesome cheat meals to help you with the compliance bit, so I've no doubt you'll love the program once you find your feet with it.

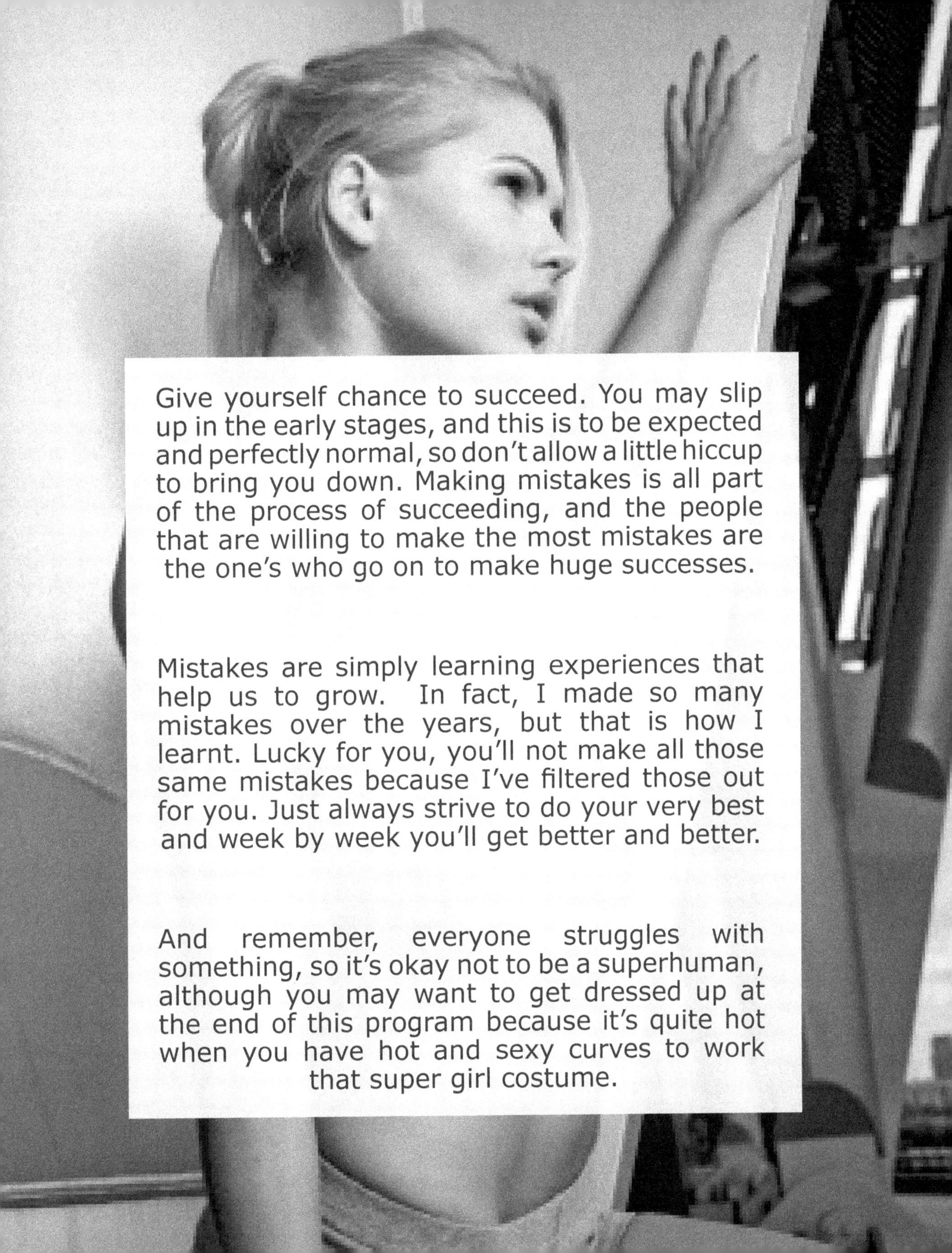

Give yourself chance to succeed. You may slip up in the early stages, and this is to be expected and perfectly normal, so don't allow a little hiccup to bring you down. Making mistakes is all part of the process of succeeding, and the people that are willing to make the most mistakes are the one's who go on to make huge successes.

Mistakes are simply learning experiences that help us to grow. In fact, I made so many mistakes over the years, but that is how I learnt. Lucky for you, you'll not make all those same mistakes because I've filtered those out for you. Just always strive to do your very best and week by week you'll get better and better.

And remember, everyone struggles with something, so it's okay not to be a superhuman, although you may want to get dressed up at the end of this program because it's quite hot when you have hot and sexy curves to work that super girl costume.

IT'S TIME

TO BUILD THE

HOTTEST CURVES

EVER

SO, SEE YOU ON THE

OTHER SIDE...

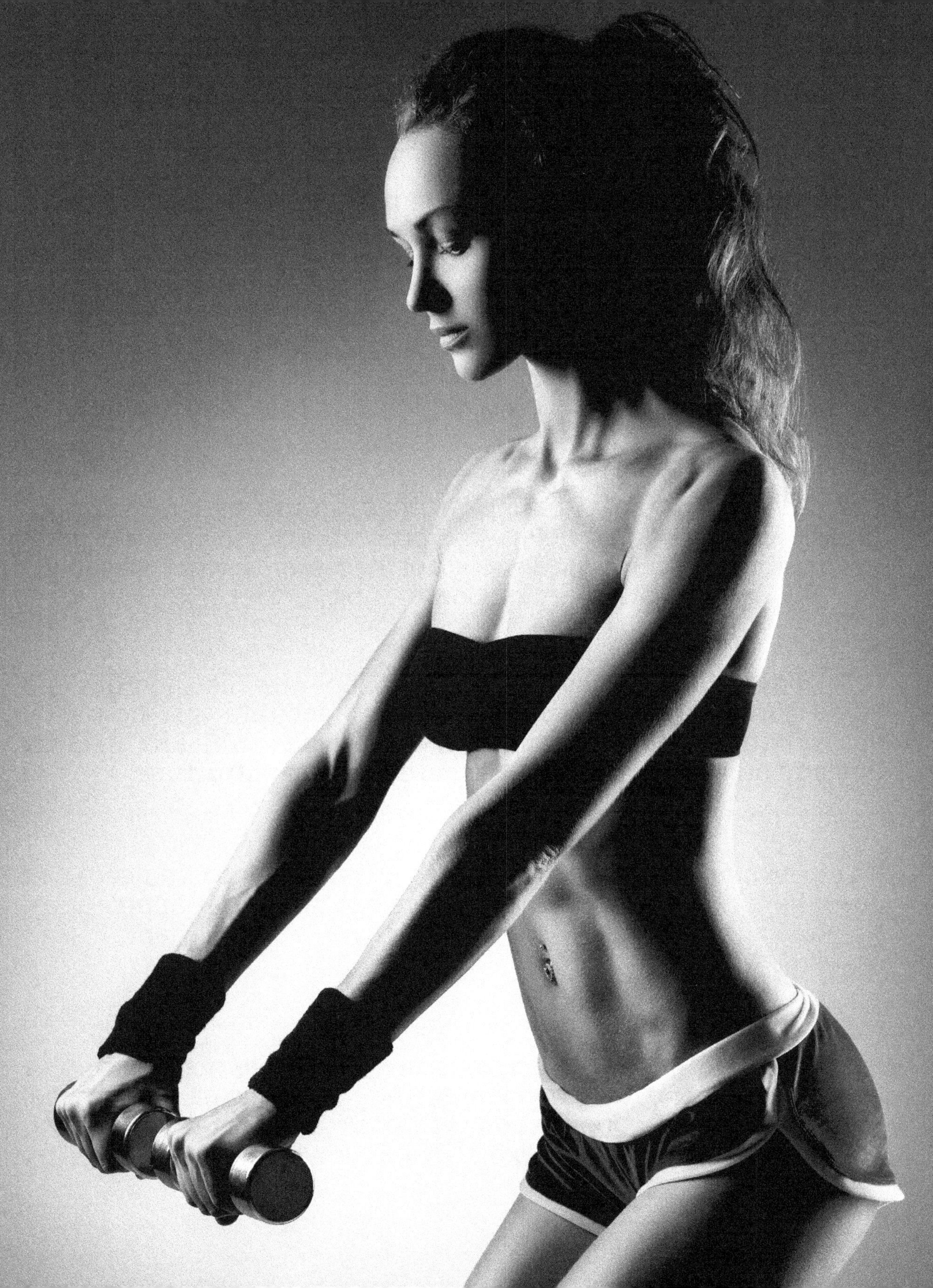

the fine art of BODY RECOMPOSITION

Skinny fat is a horrible place to be. Most females will confuse their soft exterior with being fat and run straight for fat loss programs. Yes fat loss will be necessary to achieve a tight and toned body, however, there is a difference between being fat and being soft, and this is where the confusion lies and frustration occurs.

Unfortunately, there are a lot of fitness guru's that mistakingly prescribe conventional weight loss programs to us skinny fat gals, not realising that weight loss is not necessarily what we need. Allow me to elaborate a bit further.

Your body composition is a vital component in achieving tight and toned curves. The images opposite demonstrate just how vital this is. Both ladies are obviously slim, but you can clearly see that the lady on the right has much more muscular structure.

If you have a low level of muscle mass, you're going to have to diet down hard and get super lean to lose the skinny fat appearance. As you can imagine, this is not healthy, it's not fun and it isn't sustainable.

Worse still, because you lack muscle, you'll have nothing to give you the shape and definition you are aiming for, so all you'll reveal after all that hard work is a bony structure that leaves you looking frail and starved. Ugh, not exactly what you had in mind I'm sure.

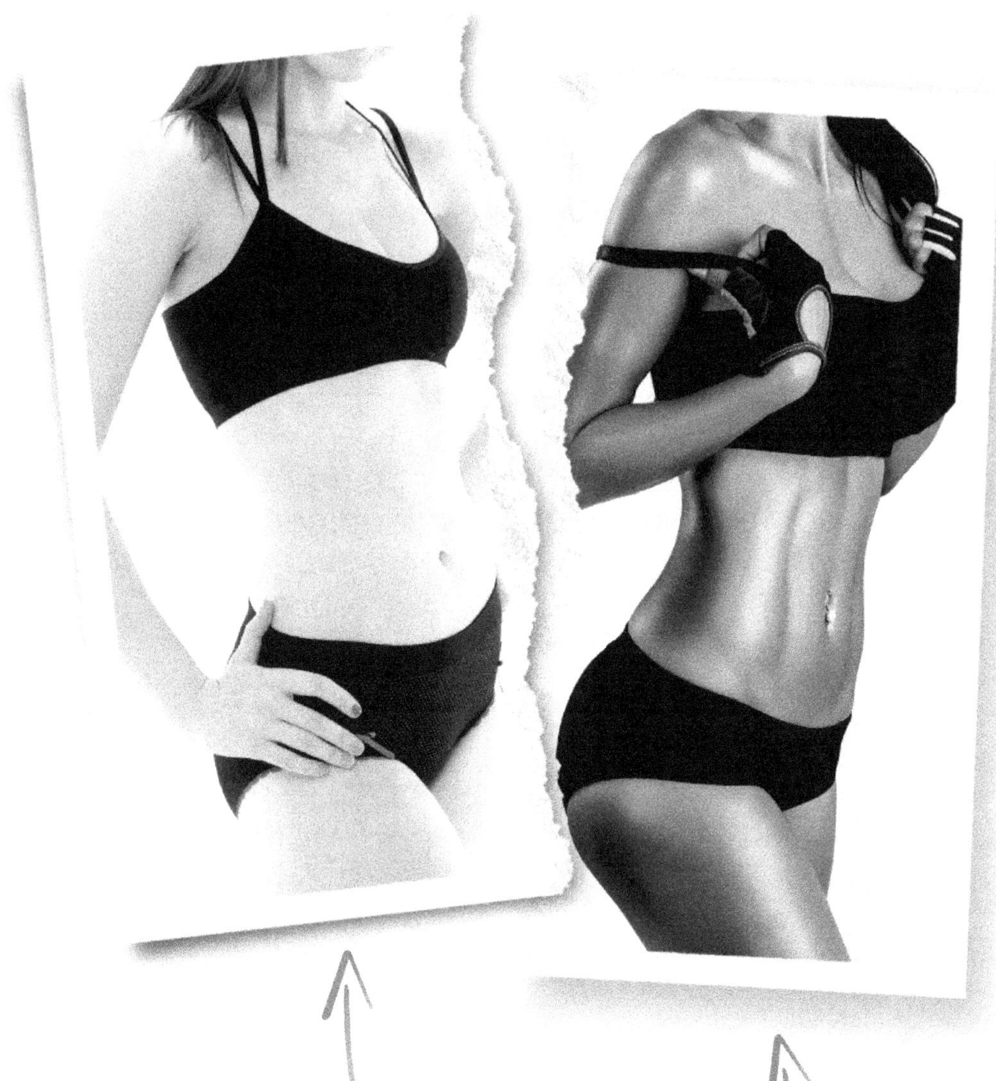

Conventional weight loss
Body recomp

Your butt will look far better too

The shape of your butt is directly related to the strength of your glutes. Weak, unused, neglected glutes are going to give you a saggy and flat butt, that lacks depth and fullness. A pair of glutes that are in shape, strengthened and well trained, however, will look very different. They will be perky, round and shapely. And what is the ultimate difference between the two? Muscle. It's all about muscle.

And there are many more upsides to increasing your muscle mass. Muscle is very metabolic, meaning that you'll burn more calories and have an easier time dropping fat. Better still, if you do put on some fat through over indulgences, which we all do once in a while, muscle looks great even with a few fatty pounds covering it. It's a win-win.

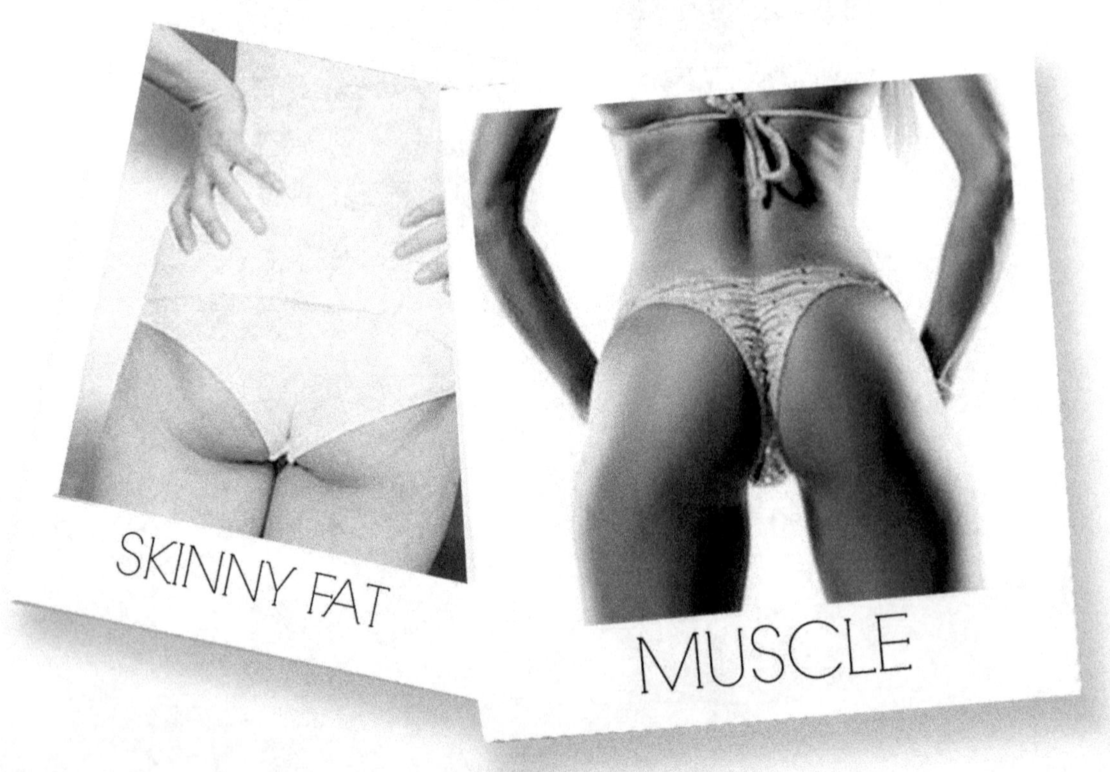

THE PROBLEMS WITH CARDIO

Here are just some of the problems with cardio:

+ Long sessions are counterproductive to muscle growth
+ Too much cardio leads to muscle loss
+ Cardio can stress the body, leading to weight gain and muffin top
+ Cardio makes you hungry, which may lead to eating back the calories burned
+ The body adapts to increase efficiency, resulting in less calories being burned

WHY TRAINING?

Weight training, on the other hand, is a body composition and sculpting tool which, conveniently, also includes all the fat loss benefits of cardio exercise. However, weight training has benefits far and beyond those gained from cardio. Let's take a brief look at some of those.

+ Improvements in body composition means a leaner and tighter body

+ Targeted weight training causes changes in body shape and enhances feminine curves

+ More muscle mass means increased resting metabolic rate

+ An increased metabolic rate means maintenance is easier

+ Weight training increases calorie burn post training

+ Heavy lifting burns more energy, making it effective for fat loss

+Weightlifting helps preserve lean mass while restricting calories for fat loss

+ Posture is lifted

+ Cellulite diminished

And much more besides

So, going back to the cardio vs weight training debate. Cardio exercise is a great fat loss tool when used correctly and in conjunction with a structured weight training program. However, if your goal is to carve out a tight and toned bikini body with plenty of sexy curves, then cardio exercise is better used as a supplement to weight training, not the primary focus.

When it comes to body composition, there is such a thing as too much cardio, so the key is to use it in a way that minimises muscle loss and maximises fat loss.

How much cardio you need is ultimately determined by how lean you are, how lean you are looking to get, and your genetics.

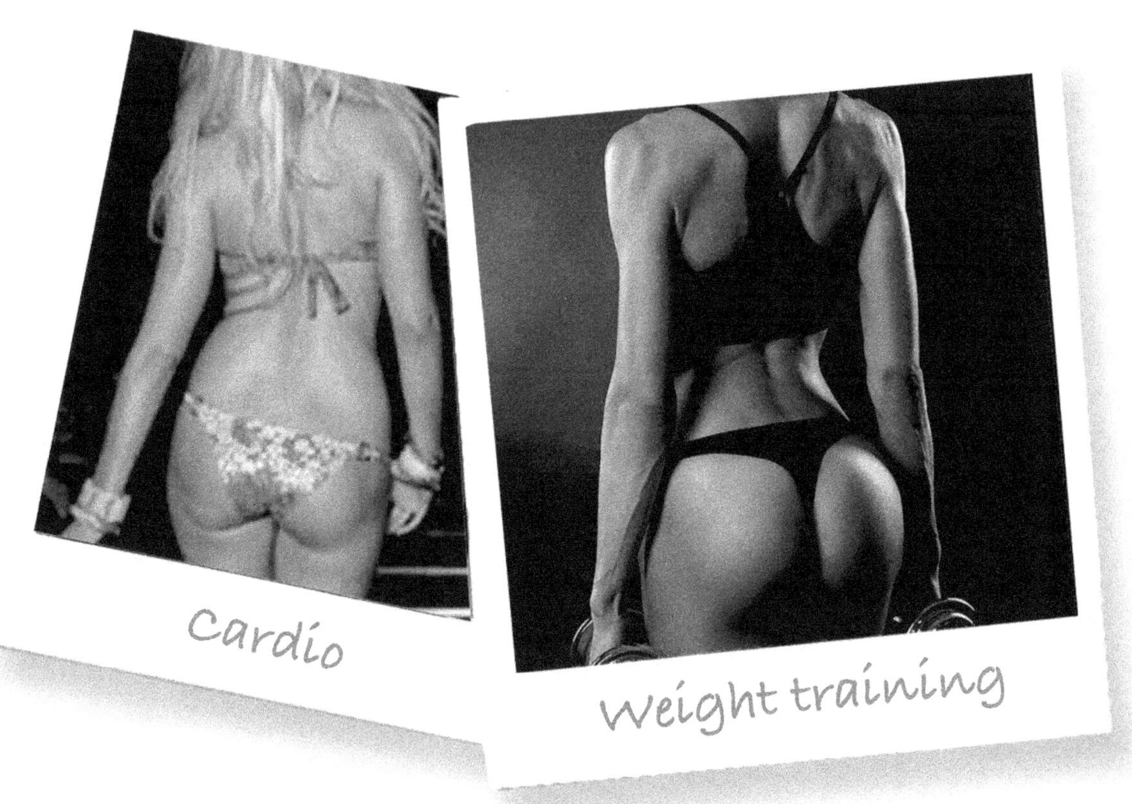

WEIGHT TRAINING VERSUS CARDIO

Have you ever noticed how many people slog away on the cardio machines in the gym, or take every aerobics class available? And yet have you also noticed how their bodies never seem to change? Unfortunately, these people are just following the age old flawed advice of doing lots of cardio to lose weight.

I'm not having a dig here because I was one of them once upon a time. At my peak, I was running a minimum of 5 miles a day, even suffering through painful shin splints. Eventually I started adding in extra HIIT sessions for good measure, and even some occasional 10 milers. I thought I was gonna be hot stuff. Sure I had a solid level of fitness, but little did I realise that I was only fuelling my skinny fat cycle.

I'm not saying cardio is bad or wrong. The problem is, many people don't understand the concept of body composition, and they certainly don't understand how to use cardio in the right way.

THE DEADLY COMBO

When trying to reduce body fat, most people increase cardio and lower their calories. When you're in a caloric deficit, your body is already primed for muscle loss. Add to this low carbs and cardio on an empty stomach and say goodbye to your beautiful muscle and hello skinny fat syndrome.

How does this happen?

Well, after a certain point, energy from your food becomes exhausted. At this point your body seeks a new source of energy to maintain it's requirements and keep you moving. Sure, part of this supply is from fat storage, but it also begins to metabolise your muscle along with it. Worse still, in a drastic caloric deficit, the body shifts to starvation mode. This is where fat is spared for life preservation, and muscle is shed because it is calorie consuming. At this point, the weight loss you see reflected back on the scales is partially at the expense of precious muscle.

When working on fat reduction, some muscle loss is inevitable, so the goal is to maintain as much lean mass and strength as possible, while maximising fat burning. There are four key elements that will help you offset the muscle burn effect as you reduce your fat storage:

+ Reduce cardio to shorter and more intense HIIT sessions
+ Supplement with Amino's or BCAA drink before or during cardio
+ Retain only a moderate caloric deficit
+ Maintain adequate protein intake
+ Focus on lifting heavy weights first and foremost

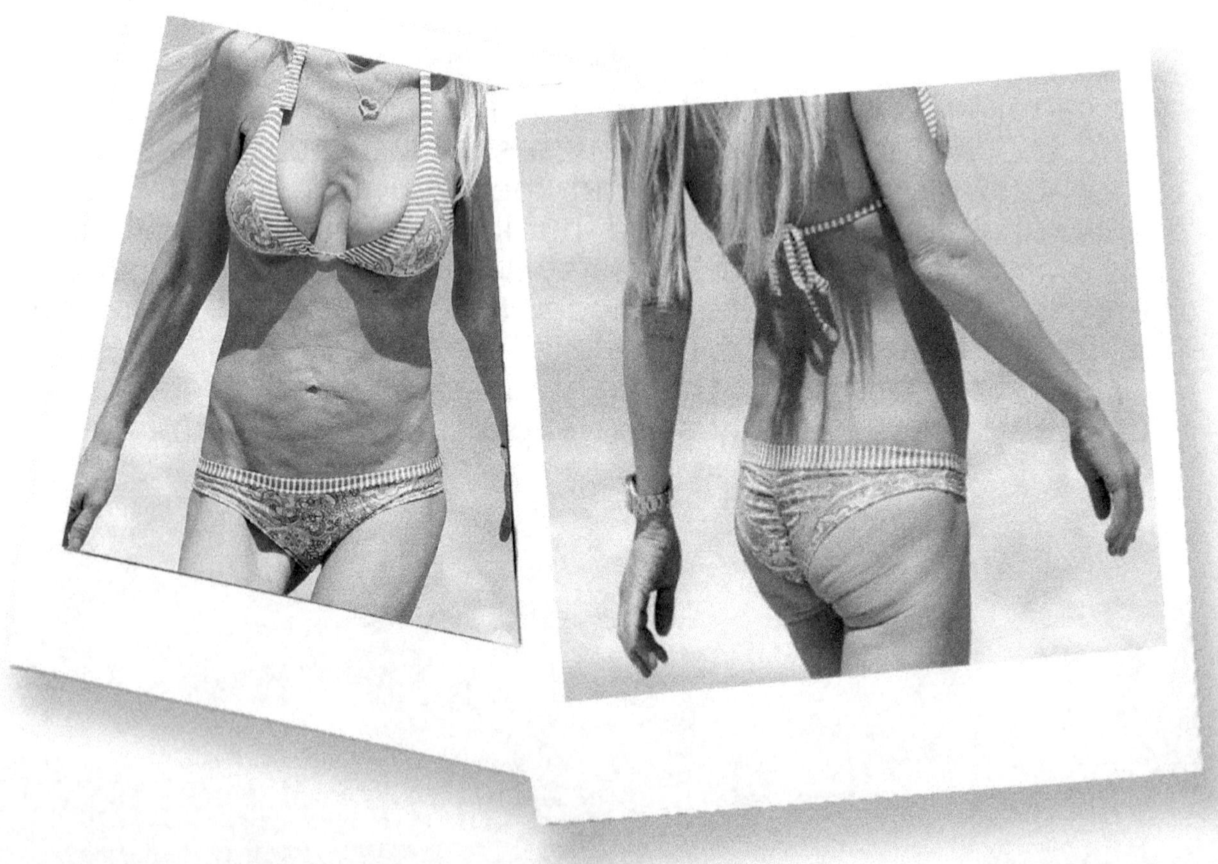

ADDRESSING COMMON CONCERNS

Body recomposition can seem like a scary process because there are far too many misunderstandings and flawed approaches circulating that have put females off weight training. Going through a successful body recomposition process requires ignoring advice given by mainstream media and some fitness gurus, and being willing to start over with a fresh perspective.

In particular, you're going to have to ditch your reliance on the scales and alter your view on weight lifting and developing muscles because here's the bottom line... Whatever your genetics, if you want to totally transform your body from skinny fat to tight and toned, you need to build muscle and, in order to build muscle, you need to lift heavy weights. It's that simple.

So, with that said, let's take a loot at the common concerns women have about the process and dispel the misconceptions .

GETTING BULKY

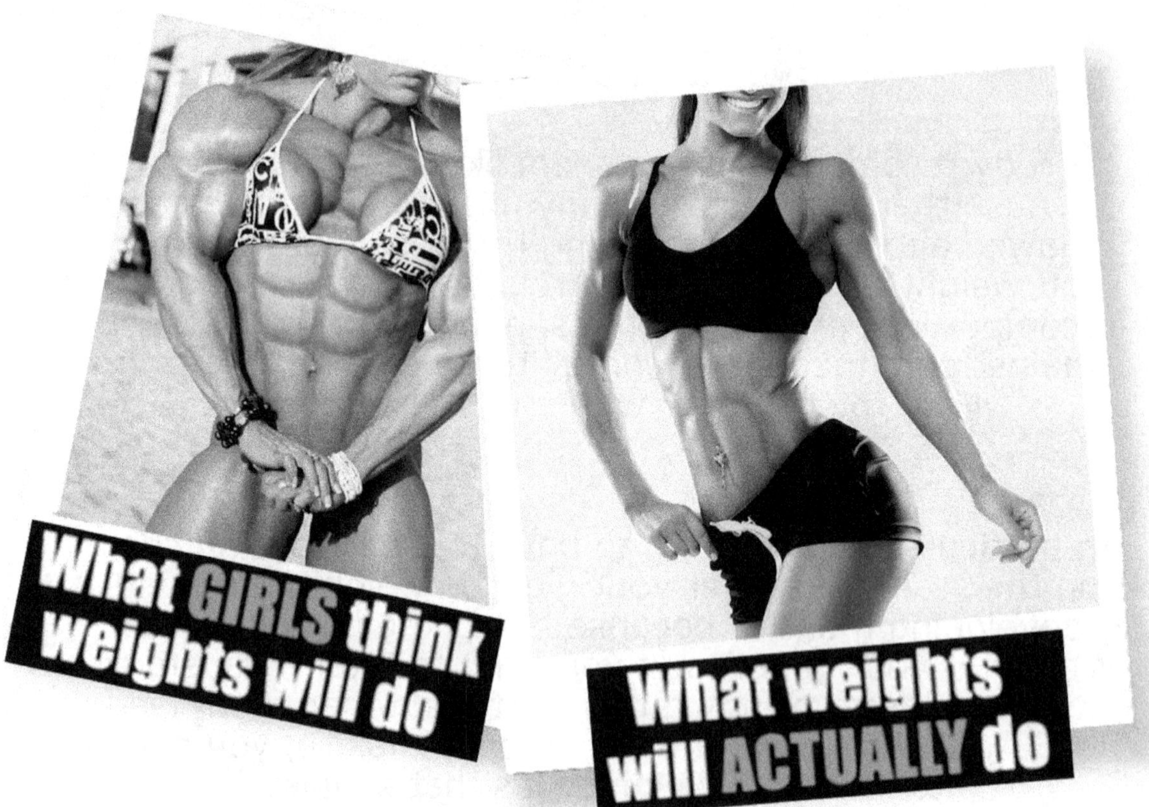

If you are afraid of lifting heavy weights because you fear getting too big and bulky, let me clarify your concerns.

I'll be honest with you. Getting bulky is a real and completely logical concern. It is entirely possible to get bulky if you follow mindless muscle building programs that pick out a list of exercises and machines, without regard for your individual body shape and the outcome being created. The DreamCurves™ program is not one of those.

DreamCurves™ is highly researched and you will work on developing your whole body, with the emphasis on creating balanced and streamlined proportions. Within our programs, we will teach you what exercises will work best for you and what exercises to avoid, resulting in some very sexy and feminine curves that are in proportion to your body shape.

As for getting too big, most people don't realise the shear amount of work that goes into getting big, let alone the fact that us females just aren't genetically built to gain lots of muscular size without the use of synthetic enhancements.

The images you see of muscle bound women is the result of several hours of training per day, years of hard work and some use of enhancements. But don't fear, I promise I'll not be promoting any such drugs on this program, and you certainly won't be training for endless hours.

Now, let's say for arguments sake that you're a genetically superior miracle who does grow muscles like weeds. You are in control of how you use this program and that means you can also use your initiative to pull back if you so desire. In fact, I encourage you to use your initiative because I want you to learn all you can during this program. Having said that, I also want you to trust in the process and be able to distinguish between your fear versus the reality.

Here's the funny thing. As a newbie to training, your body will develop muscle a bit faster than someone accustomed to training, but that'll soon slow down and, trust me, when you discover how muscle can transform the appearance of your body for the better, you'll be pleading for them to grow faster. Getting big or bulky is not a problem with this program, unless you consider firm rounded glutes, shapely shoulders and killer legs too bulky. I sure hope not.

SCALE WEIGHT

Uh oh, I gained a pound. Gasp!!!

Okay, I'm being a little facetious there, but far too many people get so wrapped up in weight loss that they don't consider where that weight is coming from and end up losing precious lean muscle mass, thus continuing the skinny fat cycle.

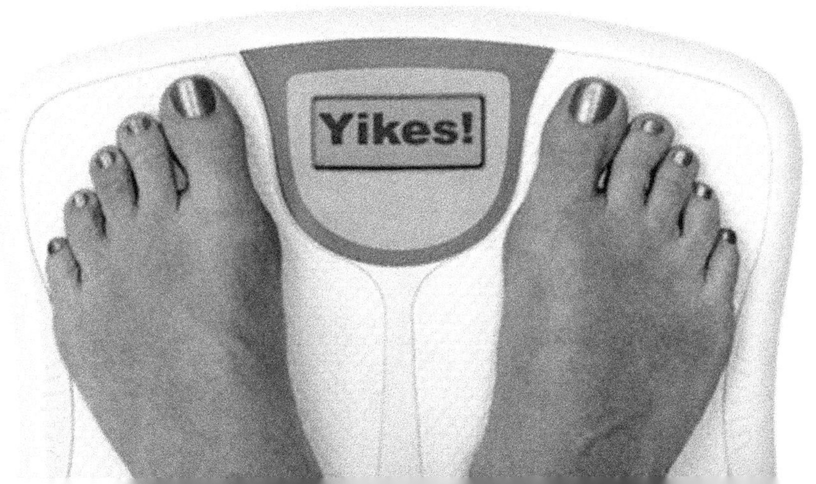

If you are worried about weight gain, now is the time to adjust that thinking because you will more than likely put on some weight during a recomposition process. Why is this? Because muscle is denser and heavier than fat, and the goal is to increase muscle, not to mention that hydration levels fluctuate daily.

This is why having some knowledge about how a body recomposition process works is crucial to your sanity.

As you begin gaining lean muscle, there may be some weeks where the number on the scales don't budge, or you may even find your weight increase slightly. If you have any hang ups on the number reflected back at you, a body recomposition process will surely be a stressful one.

Scales do have their place, and we will be using them as part of this process, however, weight gain is not something to be feared when it is coming from lean body mass. In fact, it is to be celebrated because more muscle means an increase in your metabolism and you'll burn more calories while at rest. We do use scales within this program, but we use them alongside a variety of tools so we can better understand where the progress being made.

Don't worry, you'll be rocking a super hot bikini body in no time if you trust the process.

GETTING FAT

Similarly to the fear of getting big and bulky or putting on weight, women are afraid of getting fat so they skimp on calories and wonder why they end up looking soft and skinny, with zero signs of definition.

Here's the thing, you need to eat in order to grow muscle, so the key is to eat and train correctly and consistently so that those calories are used to build your muscles and are not converted to excess fat storage.

Some of the ways this can be achieved is by following these guidelines:

+ Train heavy and often to increase insulin sensitivity
+ Introduce some high rep training days to keep your heart rate elevated
+ Perform some interval cardio and plyometric sessions
+ On NON-training days, reduce calories just below maintenance and lower your carbs
+ On training days, increase calories to slightly above maintenance and keep carbs around your training
+ Avoid eating to excess or overindulging on re-feed meals

MUFFIN TOP

An accumulation of fat around your waistline, better known as a muffin top, could indicate that your body is experiencing high levels of insulin release with your meals, or you are suffering from excess cortisol.

LOVE HANDLES

If you struggle with fat deposits under your shoulder blades, better know as love handles, you may have poor insulin sensitivity

If either of these hormones are the cause, these need to be addressed else you'll maintain that muffin top and love handles. So let's take a look at each of these in order.

INTRODUCE CARBS ONLY AROUND YOUR TRAINING

On training days when your energy needs are increased, introduce carbohydrates around your training where they are primed for use, especially after your training where they can replenish glycogen stores and increase protein synthesis. This is also the best time to have higher GI carbs because you'll want the insulin spike to shuttle protein to your muscle cells quickly.

LOWER CARB INTAKE ON REST DAYS

On rest days when you are mostly sedentary, your needs for energy are much lower. As such, taking a low carb day on rest days can avoid unnecessary demands for insulin production.

EAT LOW GI CARBS

Sticking to low GI carbs will slow the release of insulin

COMBINE

Eating carbohydrates in isolation will cause insulin to spike. You can reduce this effect by combining them with foods that increase insulin sensitivity. Here are some of the best additions you can make:

Vinegar increases glucose uptake by the muscle cells

Protein slows down the absorption rate of carbs

Fibre reduces absorption of carbs

Fish oils mimics insulin and enhances glucose metabolism

Cinnamon with your meals reduces fasting insulin levels and lowers glucose

Green Tea with meals, may inhibit the production of glucose, preventing blood sugar spikes

GET ACTIVE

Strength training and high intensity cardio activity demands high levels of glucose for energy. This demand utilises glucose at a faster rate, increasing glucose uptake by your muscles. This, in turn, improves insulin sensitivity as the body doesn't need to produce as much insulin to clear the glucose from the bloodstream.

This can continue for upward of 24 hours following your workout. In addition, as you increase your muscle mass, your storage capacity for glycogen also increases, thus becoming more efficient

+ Increase your muscle to increase their storage capacity
+ Perform high intensity cardio and weight train to burn glycogen stores
+ Take regular breaks and remain active

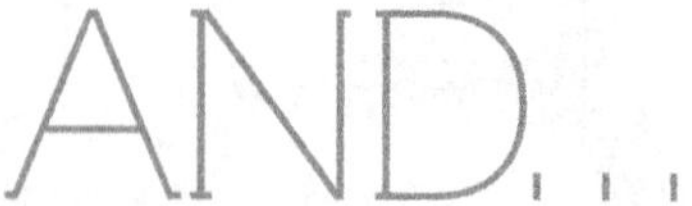

Here are some additional things you can do:

+ Avoid overindulging in high GI sugary food and drinks
+ Eat more vegetables
+ Avoid drinking large amounts of alcohol
+ Have apple cider vinegar before bed
+ Avoid liquid fructose, high fructose corn syrup and agave
+ Supplement with magnesium
+ Avoid strict dieting

Note: If you have diabetes, please seek appropriate medical advice before starting the DreamCurves or any other program.

STRESS & CORTISOL

Not only can too much cortisol lead to health problems if sustained, it can also totally ruin your beautiful hourglass shape by allowing fat to take shelter right on your curves. The good news is, while fat cannot be spot reduced, a muffin top caused by stress can be controlled.

So what is cortisol? Cortisol is a stress hormone that is released under situations of physical, mental, emotional and environmental stress. Before you close this document and declare that you are not stressed and this is not relevant to you, hear me out because there is more to stress than losing your temper with that annoying jerk who just cut you up in traffic or feeling peeved by your annoying boss.

SOME CAUSES

Stress occurs in many forms, even in those that you may not suspect, such as:

+ Exercise
+ Lack of sleep and exhaustion
+ Anxiety and depression
+ Extreme dieting and skipping meals
+ Stimulants, such as caffeine and alcohol
+ Digestive issues and inflammation
+ Bright lights and technology

Some levels of stress are perfectly fine and can even assist the body, providing extra strength and alertness. The problem occurs when stress is chronic and sustained as these can be detrimental to your health and body composition.

UNDERSTAND THE SYMPTOMS

After a stress induced cycle, blood sugar levels can plummet and crash, leaving you craving sugar and stimulants. So, next time you find yourself craving something sweet or feel like you need a boost, it could be due to stress. Drink water, go for a short walk, use deep breathing exercises and relaxation techniques and see if the cravings subside. Fuelling up on sugar or stimulants will only continue the cycle.

BEWARE OF STRESS INDUCING STIMULANTS

Caffeine releases adrenaline and, therefore, stress. Use in moderation and avoid if under any undue stress. Caffeine can be found in chocolate, fizzy pop, tea, and coffee.

Alcohol is another stimulant that increases stress levels, so reduce and moderate consumption.

BOWEL MOVEMENTS

When constipation occurs, all sorts of bacteria and waste products are left permeating in the gut, fats and toxins cannot be eliminated efficiently and re-enter circulation. In this case, liver becomes backed up with waste material, inflammation occurs, which leads to abdominal swelling.

FIBRE

Fibre is important for bowel movements, however, if your diet has been lacking in the fibre department for quite some time, your body may not be able to correctly assimilate a substantial increase straight away, which can make your bloating problems even worse. So the key is to increase your fibre intake gradually.

You can do this by spacing fibrous foods and supplements gradually through the day in increasing portions as your body becomes accustomed.

If you don't do much in the evening, you can also make the most of this alone time by experimenting with larger portions when no one is around to notice any bloating.

FLUID

Insufficient water intake leads to dehydration, which leads to constipation. Just like fibre, if your intake is increased dramatically overnight, your body kinda freaks out and could start to retain it, making you appear puffy and adding to the bloated feeling. Again, the key is to space your intake gradually throughout the day, and avoid drinking excessive amounts with your meals when it can hamper digestion.

COLON CLEANSE & MAGNESIUM

If you have suffered from constipation, magnesium may help to relax your intestines for easier passage. Alternatively you can try a natural colon cleansing product, such as Oxy-Powder® which will help clear any impaction. Just be sure to take it according to the instructions and at a time when you are going to be at home close to the toilet as it is very very powerful.

If you're changing some of your eating habits, your body may be lacking the enzymes it needs to process some of the nutrients, and it's not uncommon to experience some digestion problems that cause bloating and gas during the transition. This is where a natural digestive enzyme supplement can assist.

I recommended taking an enzyme formula whenever you introduce a new whole food, and taper them off over time as the bloating subsides and your body adapts.

LACK OF SALT

Insufficient sea salt intake can have a negative impact on your digestive health. This is because salt produces hydrochloric acid (HCL) in your stomach which creates stomach acid. Stomach acid is needed to digest food.

TAKE IT SLOW

Gradual changes and introductions can be better for your gut than abrupt shifts in eating habits, so take it slow and let your body adapt at it's pace. At least when you introduce new foods one by one you can see what the reaction is and can effectively deal with it.

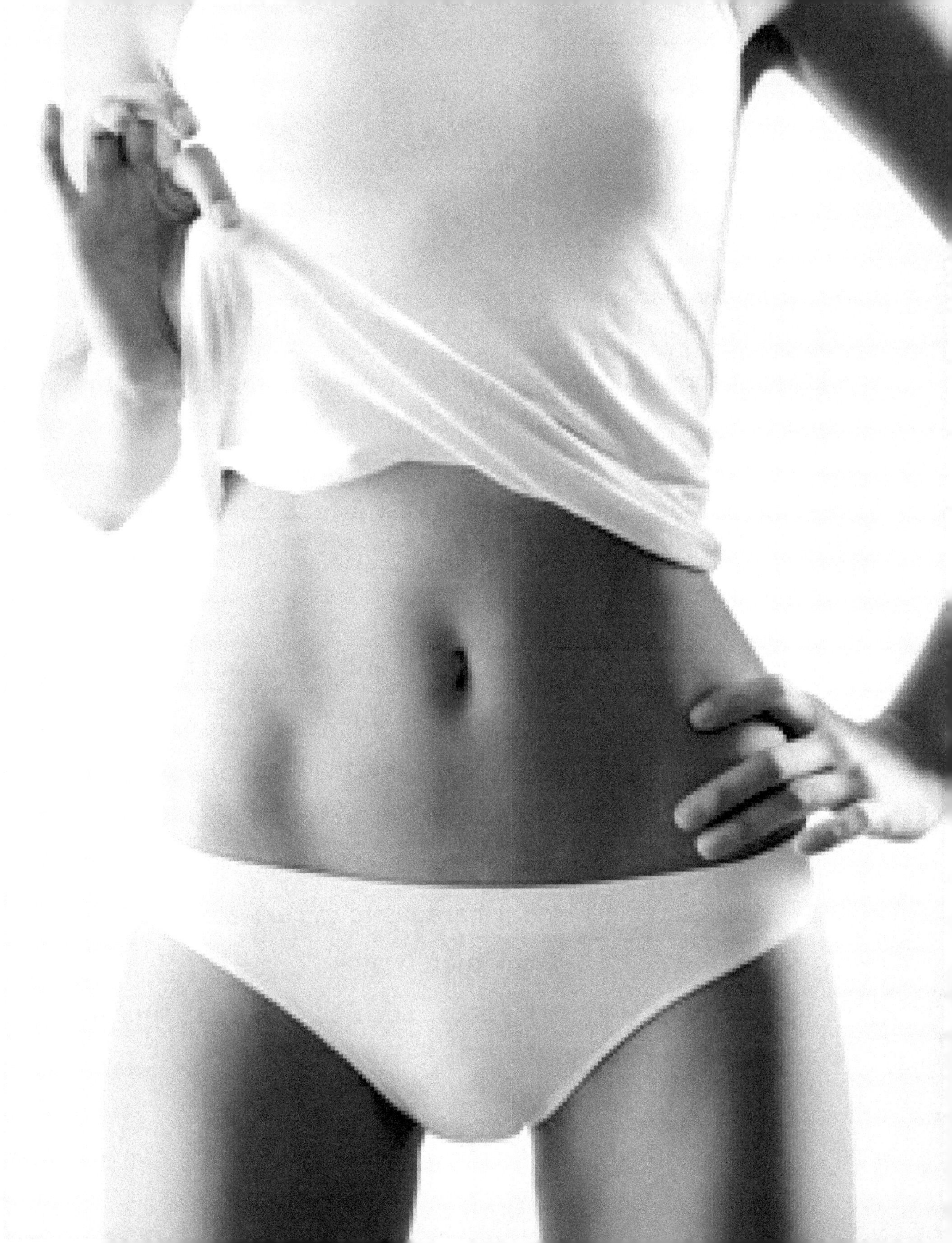

FLUID RETENTION

An often overlooked and unexpected cause of bloating and water retention is salt. Too much salt will bind to water and cause water retention and bloating, while conversely so too will insufficient amounts as you body will become dehydrated and store water for survival.

Be cautious about how much salt you add to your meals, and be especially careful about prepackaged foods. Here are some guidelines:

+ Limit consumption of canned and preserved foods
+ Avoid processed meats
+ Reduce salt on your meals
+ Use Himalayan sea salt in place of table salt
+ Stick to low sodium dressings
+ Eat celery and asparagus to expel water
+ Drink more water
+ Include potassium rich foods, such as bananas, squash, and salmon

GASEOUS FOODS

There are some foods which are known to cause flatulence and contribute to a gassy and bloated stomach . If you suffer form bloating, you'll want to limit these problematic foods as much as possible or take in smaller amounts while you body adapts. Some of these are:

+ Foods high in sugar. Sugar ferments in the gut and contributes to candida and inflammation
+ Dairy products, including processed and high sugar yogurts
+ Beans and legumes.
+ Cabbage, Brussel sprouts, broccoli and cauliflower
+ Refined grains and gluten
+ Carbonated beverages

You may also find artificial sweeteners and sugar alcohols problematic, such as aspartame, sorbitol, xylitol, Sucralose etc. Even chewing gum can cause problems.

BACTERIA

Bacteria overgrowth is when the bad bacteria in your intestines outweigh the good bacteria. If you defences are down, all hell breaks loose right there on your waistline and you'll need to bring in some reinforcements to increase your levels of beneficial bacteria. You can do this by pro-biotic supplementation or foods containing high levels of good bacteria, such as yogurt. It is absolutely imperative that you select a Pro Biotic Supplement that is high potency and of the multi-strain variety.

If you have had an imbalance in your gut bacteria for a while or if it remains untreated, candida overgrowth can ensue, damaging your defences further and leading onto a whole host of even more serious problems . There are several things that contribute to candida overgrowth, these are:

+ Sugar consumption (including refined carbohydrates)
+ Oral contraceptives
+ Alcohol consumption
+ Fermented foods
+ Stress
+ Food sensitivities

The most common symptoms of candida overgrowth are:

+ Fungal infections such as athletes foot and ring worm
+ Digestive issues, bloating, constipation and diarrhoea
+ Skin problems, such as eczema and psoriasis
+ Vaginal infections and itching
+ Sugar cravings

If you think you are suffering from candida overgrowth, you'll need to carry out a candida detox and cleanse which generally involves:

+ Eliminate foods that feed candida
+ Kill off the yeast infection
+ Restores healthy bacteria levels

Unfortunately, the treatment for candida is beyond the scope of this program, and I highly recommend you seek guidance of an appropriate professional if you suffer form any of the above symptoms.

INFLAMMATION

Inflammation in your gut caused by food will affect your whole system and you'll need to seek appropriate professional guidance.

The most common and identifiable symptoms of inflammation are:

+ Severe or chronic abdominal pain
+ Digestive issues, bloating and diarrhoea (sometimes bloody)
+ Sudden weight loss
+ Lack of appetite
+ Rectal bleeding

If you have any of these symptoms, please see you doctor or a registered dietician and discontinue the use of this program.

EFFECTIVE FAT REDUCTION

So now that we've covered how a body recomposition process works and other factors which may be contributing to fat accumulation in your abdominal region, we're ready to delve into the subject of fat loss.

Unlike other flawed and faulty fitness programs you see on the market, which don't care if weight is coming from fat, muscle or water, and don't care if your metabolism is hampered in the process, I'm going to show you how to effectively reduce body fat, while maintaining your muscle mass and keeping your metabolism fired up throughout the entire process.

But first, let's take a quick look at why traditional approaches fail and leave unsuspecting participants stuck in the cycle of skinny fat syndrome.

THE BAD APPROACH

Most approaches to fat loss begin with a calorie restriction, so let's take a look at what happens in a typical calorie restricted cycle.

When you restrict your calorie intake your body fat stores will reduce, however, after some time your metabolic rate slows and so does the rate of fat loss. This is referred to as metabolic down-regulation. This happens because the less body fat you have, the more your body will attempt to hold onto those fat stores, this is just how our body's survival mechanism works

The problem with most programs is that they have you on a very restricted amount of calories which makes this down-regulation happen much faster. Then, when fat loss slows, it is typical for people to reduce their calories further, seems logical right. Well, as your body has already down-regulated your metabolism, reducing calories further not only serves to promote a further down-regulation, your body will start to enter starvation mode in order to prepare for potential famine. The more severe the calorie restriction, the more your body down-regulates, the less fat your lose and... you get my point.

It's a vicious cycle, but that's not all. Your body is super smart and, in this state, your body will start to break down muscle tissue as it's preferred source of energy. Why? Because muscle burns more calories than fat, and your body is now in preservation mode and muscle is a threat. Now when you weigh yourself, muscle wasting is typically what's reflected in the weight lost and the skinny fat cycle has begun.

Unfortunately, it gets worse.

As you're aware, most people don't stop at a simple calorie reduction for fat loss, nooooo, they add hours of gruelling cardio into the mix, unaware of the damage and devastation they are causing their body. This is where things turn especially messy. Cardio itself is not the problem, cardio while in a severe calorie deficit is the problem because your body is already in a compromised and muscle wasting state.

Adding cardio in this instance is just counterproductive as your body will use muscle for fuel to sustain it's energy requirements during the activity, as well as further down-regulating your metabolism to hold onto the body fat you still have.

And if that's not yet bad enough, there's also the addition of fad dieting principles to contend with too. Yikes. In the 80's it was low fat, today the media has just made everyone afraid to eat at all. Fats and carbs are seen as fattening and protein makes you too big. It's all BS. Without going into too much detail and causing your brain to down-regulate, let's just say that it's a vicious downward spiral from this point and you could do your body a lot of long term damage, both at a metabolic level and a hormonal one.

In essence:

A severe calorie deficit
+ long cardio sessions
+ inadequate nutrition
= **recipe for metabolic disaster**

MODERATE CALORIE DEFICIT

Use the Harris-Benedict formula to determine your baseline calories. This formula is one of the most accurate, so is the very best starting point for determining your deficit.

Many programs and online calculators underestimate how many calories you need, so any deficit on top of this already low number is just far too severe.

In order to bring your body fat levels down, I suggest using a small to moderate calorie deficit of between 15-25% below maintenance, and you'll be using the deficit on a rotation basis where they will be higher on training days than on rest days.

This means that those calories will be partitioned where they will be used and not stored.

CARBOHYDRATE MANIPULATION

As carbohydrates can inhibit your body from using fat for fuel, I also suggest manipulating their intake so that they too are partitioned where they will be useful and not inhibiting.

As with your calories, you'll be using a rotation method so that they are higher on your training days. I recommend 20% complex carbs on training days and only vegetable carbs on non-training days during the fat loss phase.

And, in addition to this cycling method, time your carbs round your training.

REFEED (CHEAT) MEAL

One of the most crucial tools when you are in a calorie deficit is the introduction of a weekly cheat meal. A cheat meal will keep your fat burning hormones high and your body from panicking itself into starvation mode. Plus you'll get to delve into a tasty treat every week.

SHORT CARDIO SESSIONS

I don't warrant checking in for the hamster wheel for long and boring snooze sessions 7 days a week. Instead say hello to HIIT training and say hello lean and sexy curves. You'll want to be in and out in no more than 30 minutes. That's it.

BUMP UP YOUR PROTEIN

Protein is the key to preserving your muscle and keeping your body turning to fat for its fuel. Durikng the fat burning phase, keep; yur protein to at least 50% of your daily intake.

HEAVY RESISTANCE TRAINING

One of the most overlooked tools for reducing body fat is heavy weight training. Lifting heavy weights causes your metabolic rate to skyrocket, and it'll transform your body like nobodies business. Forget low weight and high reps as they'll do nothing for your composition.

USE REVERSE DIETING

Once you have lost the body fat, what next? How do you stop the rebound effect? You use a technique called reverse dieting.

Reverse dieting is just how it sounds, you reverse the dieting process. So, where you would incrementally decrease your calories to lose the body fat and avoid hitting a plateau, now you will incrementally increase those calories back up to your maintenance to avoid putting excess body fat back on.

It's a technique used by fitness models, athletes and bodybuilders, and it's the missing link from most diet and fat loss programs.

Now you may be thinking that as long as you raise your calories back up to maintenance you wont' put on body fat, but this isn't the case and is the mistake may people make after being on a restricted program. Hence why many will pile back on the lbs.

The reason reverse dieting is so incredibly effective is because as you lose the body fat, your body downregulates your metabolism.

Because your body has adapted to those lower calories and the slower metabolism, reverse dieting allows your body to gradually adjust back up to your new maintenance.

Think about it like this, as you drop body fat and you've been in a calorie reduction, your body can easily over react when it suddenly has in influx of food in the system, and because your body fat is low by this point, it wants to store some body fat for potential famine.

Give the body what it needs, but in a controlled manner and you won't end up back at square one.

Unfortunately, the reverse dieting principle is not so simple for many people because it can be percieved as being more difficult than losing the body fat. The reason for this is that when you go into a reverse diet phase, your body is at a condition you are happy with, so all you want to do is tuck into a normal diet

RESIST THE URGE TO RETURN TO OLD HABITS

If you can resist the temptation to revert to old habits and see the reverse diet through, and you will reap the long term rewards. You'll not only maintain your new beautiful lean body, but you'll also avoid damaging your metabolism and will keep your hormones balanced.

If you have been on a 20 & 25% calorie deficit, start by reducing that deficit to 15 & 20% levels for 1 to 2 weeks. Keep your weekly cheat meal too. After this 1-2 weeks, reduce your calorie deficit further to the 10 & 15% mark. Do that for another 1-2 weeks. Then keep dropping the deficit every 1-2 weeks to the next increment until you hit your maintenance.

You'll also not need to continue your HIIT training, so scale that back and focus your attention on heavy weight training instead. This will prepare you to transition into the Sculpt phase where you can work on building your muscles and sculpting those sexy curves.

Once you hit maintenance calories, the level where you are not gaining or losing any more body fat. I'd suggest staying there for a few weeks to allow your body to get accustomed to not being in a deficit. Enjoy your new body for a while. Then, when you are ready, you can progress onto the sculpting your new leaner body.

12 WEEK PROGRAM

The Trim phase of this DreamCurves program is based around 12 weeks. 12 weeks is a great midddle ground that is not too restrictive, but also achieves great results in a short time frame.

However, if you have a special event coming up and really want to slim down quickly, the following page shows how to reduce the program down to 8 weeks without damaging your metabolism or hitting a plateau.

Likewise, if you would rather take a little bit longer to make the adjustments, maybe you don't want to go through so many changes at once, you can extend the Trim phase to 16 weeks, and I'll show you how to do that also.

8 WEEK ADJUSTMENTS

I don't recommend an 8 week fat loss approach simply because of the potential damage to your hormones and metabolism, however, I know that there are times when you just need to make changes ASAP and I figure if you are going to do it faster, then you should at least know how to do it using a safer approach. So here is the 8 week approach I would recommend.

The adjustments for an 8 week plan

Use the 20-25% calorie deficit range

Drop all complex carbohydrates except those in your post training meal

Have a cheat meal once a week because that will keep your metabolism high

Perform 5-6 days HIIT training, 20-30 minutes long

Perform 4-5 days resistance training, prioritise large muscle groups

You could also add 20 minutes cardio after resistance training

After 8 weeks, transition onto the standard Trim phase guidelines

Please don't attempt this 8 week program if you have just come out of an extreme diet. Your body will be compromised and you should perform a reverse diet instead.

16 WEEK ADJUSTMENTS

If you are quick happy to take a steadier approach to the fat loss phase, you can extend the phase to 16 weeks. Even with the 16 week adjustments, you'll be dropping body fat and will see incredible changes to your body, but you'll do so in a more linear and controlled way, and your body composition will benefit from a slower approach.

The adjustments for this are very simple and laid out below.

The adjustments for an 16 week plan

Use a 15% calorie deficit on both training and non-training days

Have carbs throughout the day on your training day, not just after training

MODERATE YOUR INTAKE

I'm gong to keep this section relatively brief because I'm sure you're aware that alcohol isn't the healthiest thing to consume, and I don't want to bore you or come across as being preachy.

At the end of the day, we all have our thing we consider a treat and hey, life is too short give up all those treats. However, when you're trying to reach your body transformation goals, it may help you make better choices if you understand how alcohol can effect your progress. Knowledge is power and all that good stuff.

IT'S A TOXIN

The reason alcohol is a problem for body composition is because when it is consumed it's not metabolised the same way other food and drinks are. This is because alcohol is treated as a toxin, not as nourishment. When a toxin is ingested, that toxin is immediately shuttled off to the liver to be oxidised and expelled as a matter of priority to protect your body. All other functions that are carried out by the liver are then halted while the toxin is processed. This means that the regulation and break down of body fat, which is one of the livers key functions, is hampered. As is the digestion of food and other beverages that are consumed around the same time as the alcohol, which of course puts those calorie straight to your saddlebags.

To give you an idea of just how damaging this process is, here are some facts.

It takes the liver approximately 1 hour to metabolise 1 ounce of alcohol.

At 20 ounces per pint, that a lot of down time for those other functions.

EMPTY CALORIES

Pure alcohol, without anything added, contains 7 calories per gram. This is only 2 fewer calories than fat. So, you can see that alcohol calories are dense. That's the alcohol itself without the addition of flavour, sugar and creams that are used to make it taste good. And each of those calories are empty, meaning they have no nutritional value to offer your body.

Here are some typical numbers:

Glass of Baileys = 130 calories
Pint of beer = 208 calories
Bottle of Alcopops = 171 calories

Bottoms up...

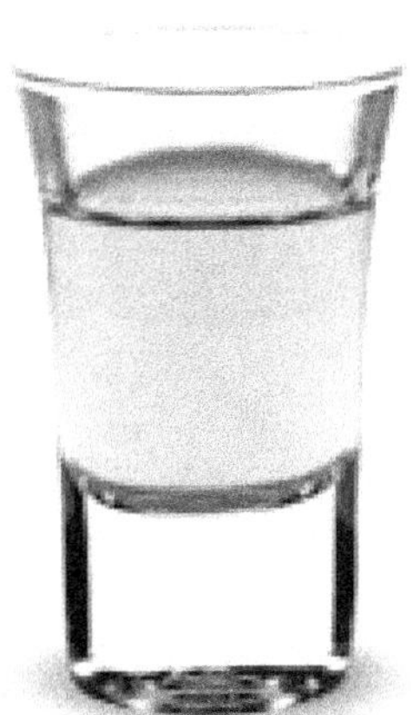

THE GOOD NEWS

Okay, so I'll leave all the bad stuff there because I'm sure you're aware of all the other problems associated with chronic alcohol intake.

The good news is that, if you're not a chronic drinker or an alcoholic, the occasional indulgence is okay and can be offset. You can also limit the effects alcohol has by mixing it up with a diet soda or tonic water. Leading a healthy lifestyle is the most important factor because any additional calories you do consume from alcohol is at least more likely to be used to fuel your activities.

The key takeaway is to limit the regularity and volume of consumption. Everything in moderation.

WHAT IS CELLULITE?

The dimpling and puckering effect associated with cellulite is caused by swollen fat cells. As you can see in the diagram above, these swollen cells put pressure on the fibrous bands, which pulls and drags the skin creating the cottage cheese effect.

The reason why a females carry cellulite and a man tends not to is due to the formation of these fibres. In a female, these fibres are distributed in vertical chambers causing the cells to bulge outward. Conversely, these fibres are denser and more mesh like in a man, causing them to expand laterally and internally. Think compression stockings covering a mans fat cells, and fishnets covering ours and you get the idea. Mother nature sure was having some fun when she came up with that one.

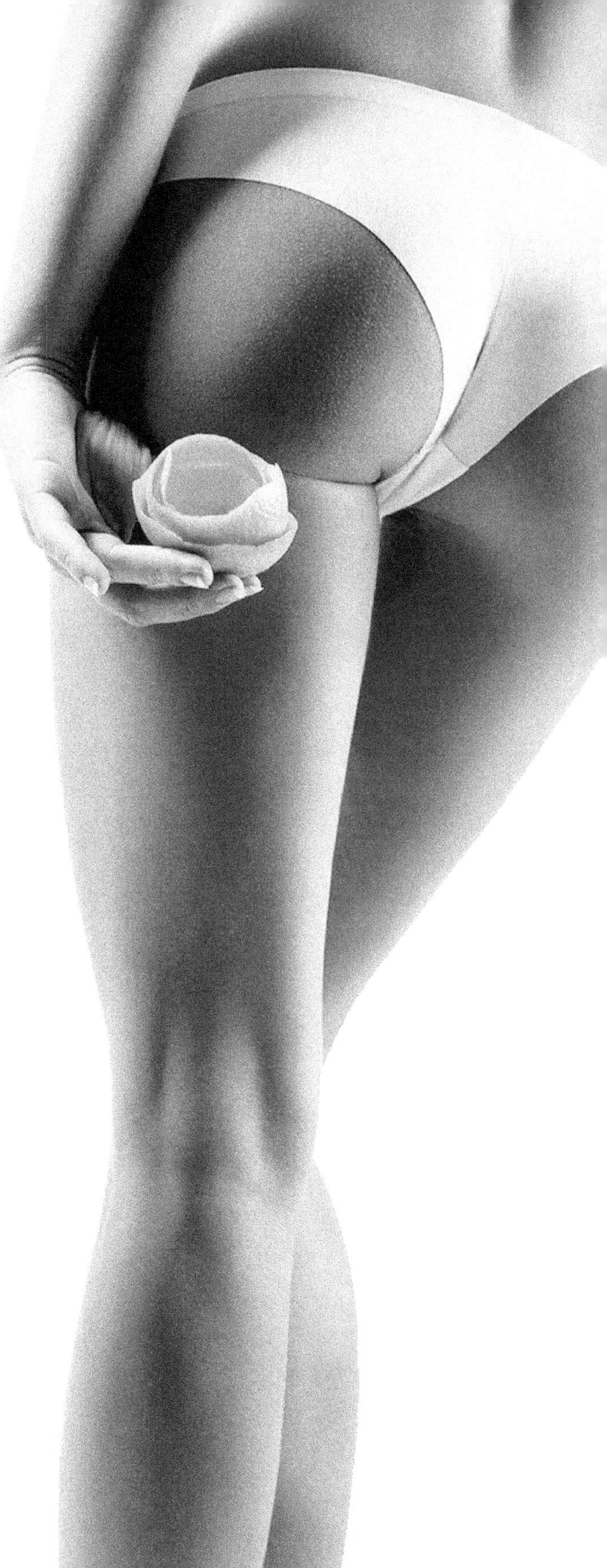

The extent to which cellulite forms on each individual is largely a factor of genetics, which is why some ladies have a harder time with it than others. As a result of these genetics, it's quite possible to see very lean individuals carrying cellulite, despite having low body fat levels and being very fit.

As we age, particularly as we enter our 30's, cellulite gets worse because our collagen production decreases, oestrogen levels drop and the cells lose their elasticity.

So, what can be done to reduce its appearance, if anything?

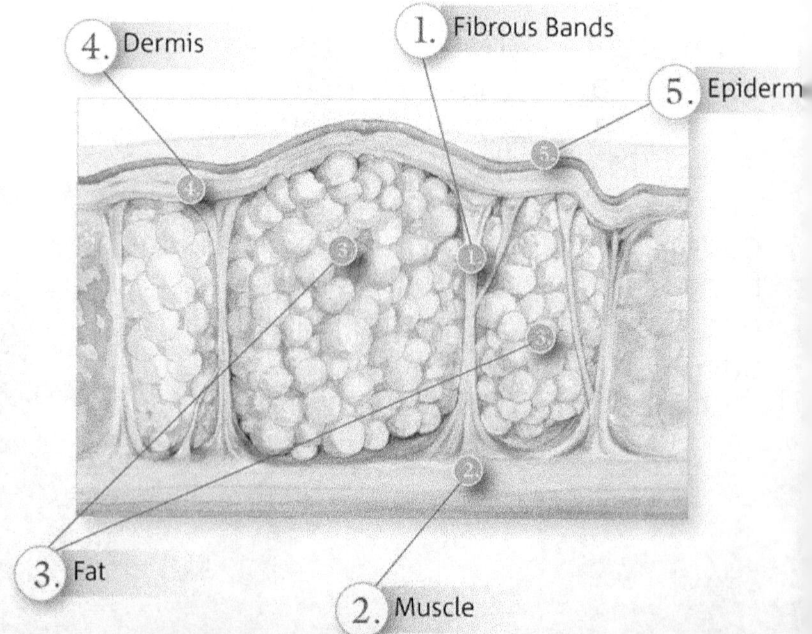

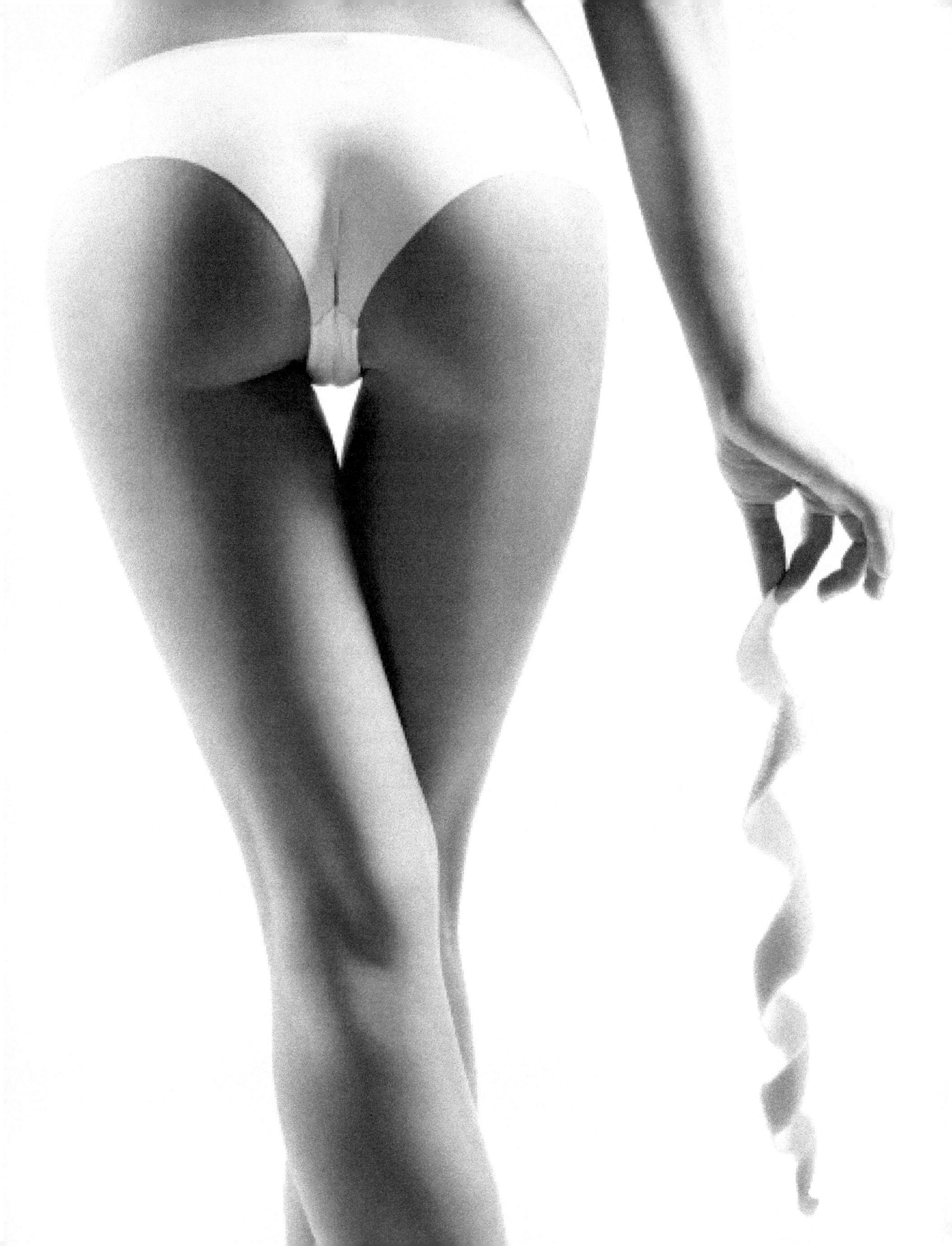

LONG TERM SOLUTIONS

Each of those things can temporarily reduce cellulite by drawing out the fluids and/or stimulating collagen production. There effects are short term, but they are quick fixes none the less that can help if you have a special occasion looming.

The treatments that work the best over the longer term involve structured exercise and nutrition. Cardio, weight training and proper nutrition are the most vital components to diminishing the unsightly appearance of cellulite in the longer term because together they work to strengthen all cells in the body, enhance blood flow, and bring balance to your hormones. Furthermore, when you lift weights, your muscles create fullness and your whole body structure tightens up, thus resulting in a smoother and tighter appearance. Proper nutrition aids digestion which reduces the build up of toxins in your fat cells, eliminates fluid retention.

Conveniently, all these factors are addressed within this program so, follow the guidelines, and cellulite reduction is all part of the service.

TASTY & NUTRITIOUS SWEET SNACKS

BANANA PORRIDGE

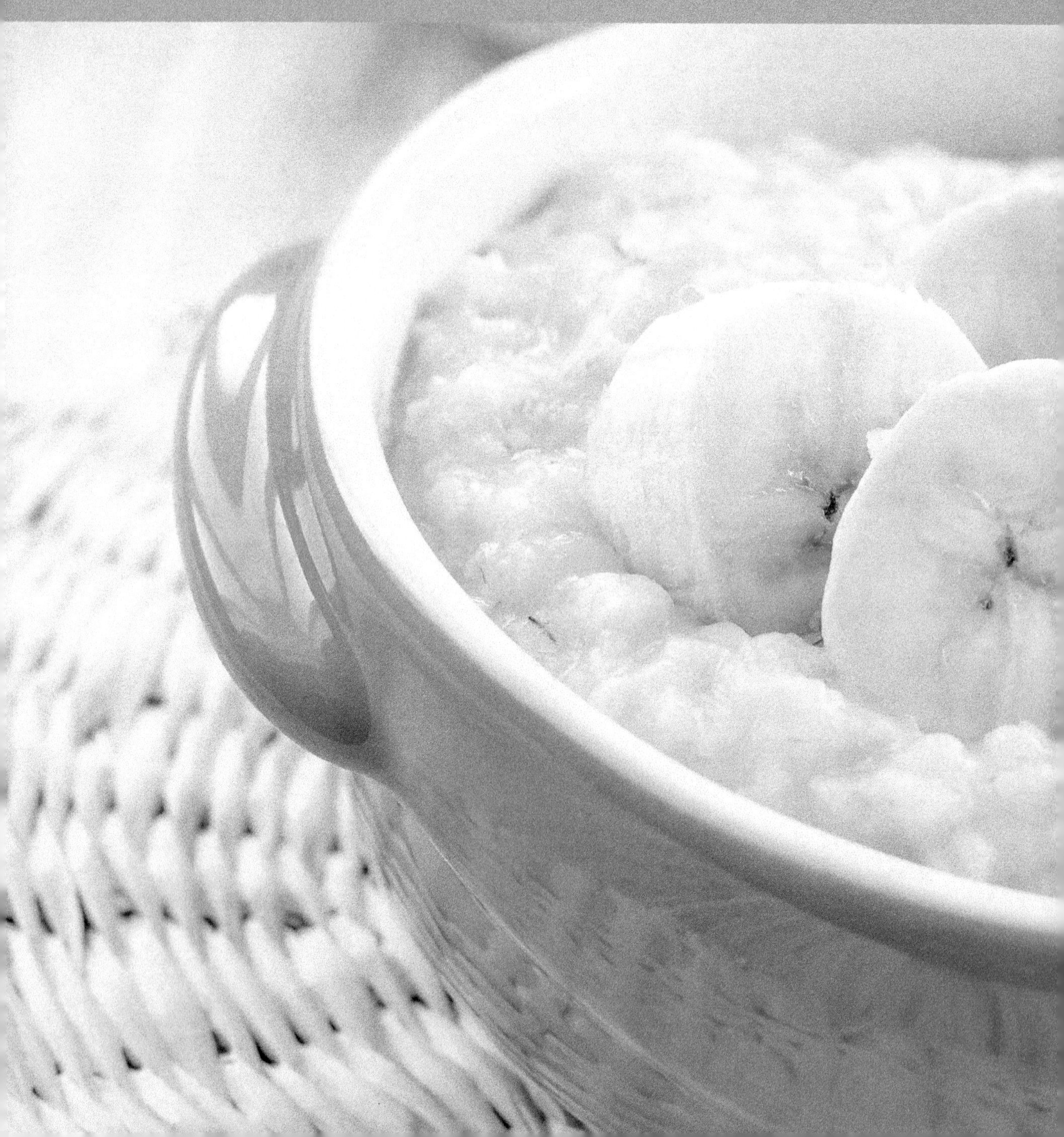

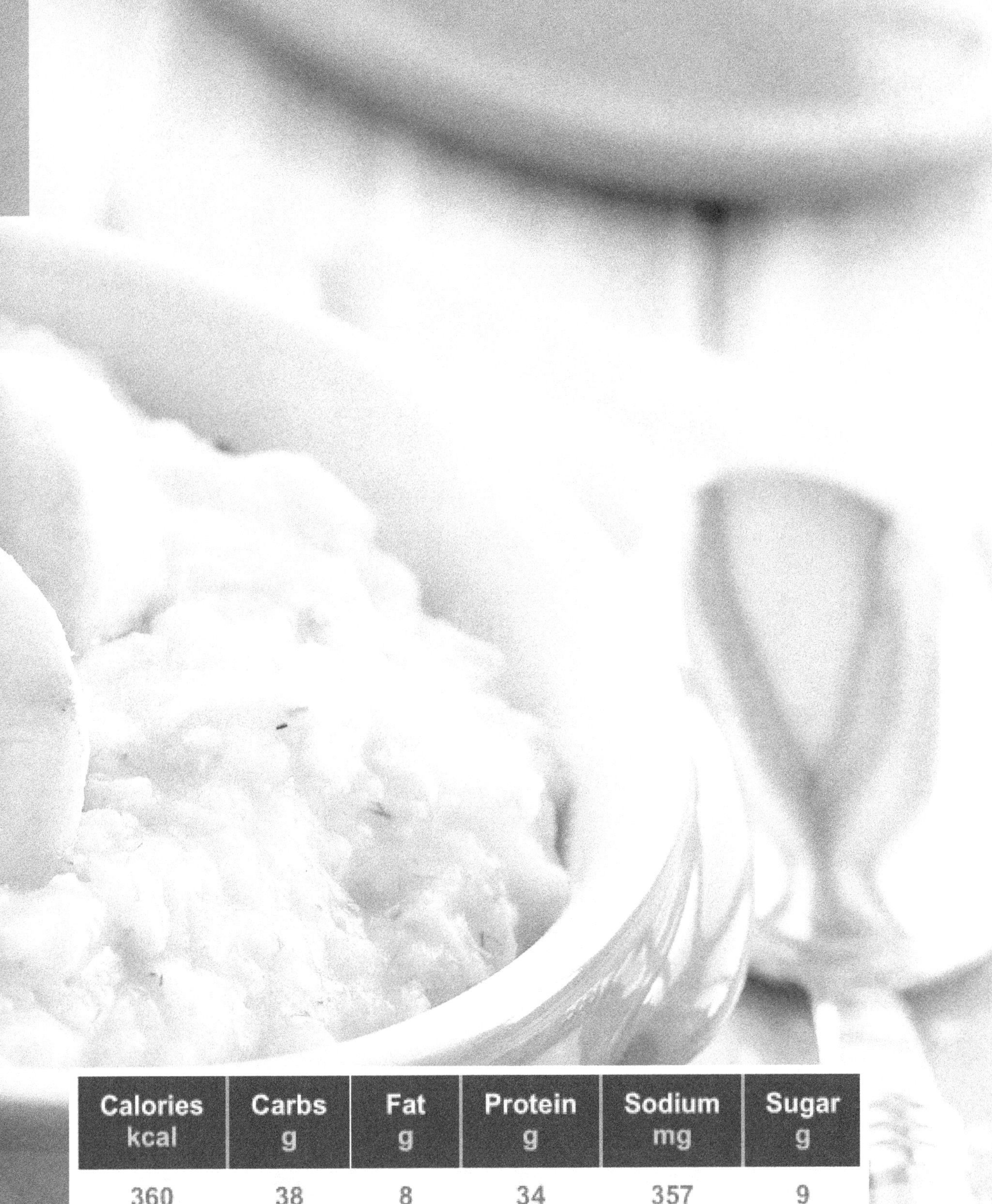

Calories kcal	Carbs g	Fat g	Protein g	Sodium mg	Sugar g
360	38	8	34	357	9

BANANA PROTEIN PORRIDGE

IDEAL POST WORKOUT SNACK 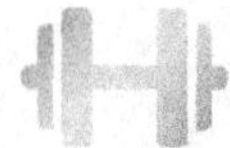

INGREDIENTS

» 1/2 cup Wholegrain Oats
» 1 cup Unsweetened Almond Milk
» 30g Whey Protein Powder (low carb) Any flavour
» 50g Banana (or fruit of choice)

Optional Extras: Stevia, Maple syrup, Honey, Himalayan sea salt, cinnamon

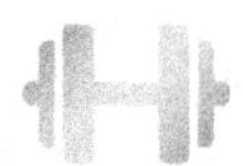 POST WORKOUT MEAL

DIRECTIONS

Bring the milk to a boil and stir in your oats. Bring back to a boil, then lower the heat and continue to cook/stir the oats until cooked (about 5-10 minutes).

Take off the heat and stir in cinnamon, and protein powder. If oatmeal is too thick for your taste, add in a little more milk until a creamy mixture forms.

Add in your optional additions, top with fruit of choice and any additional toppings.

STRAWBERRY CREPE

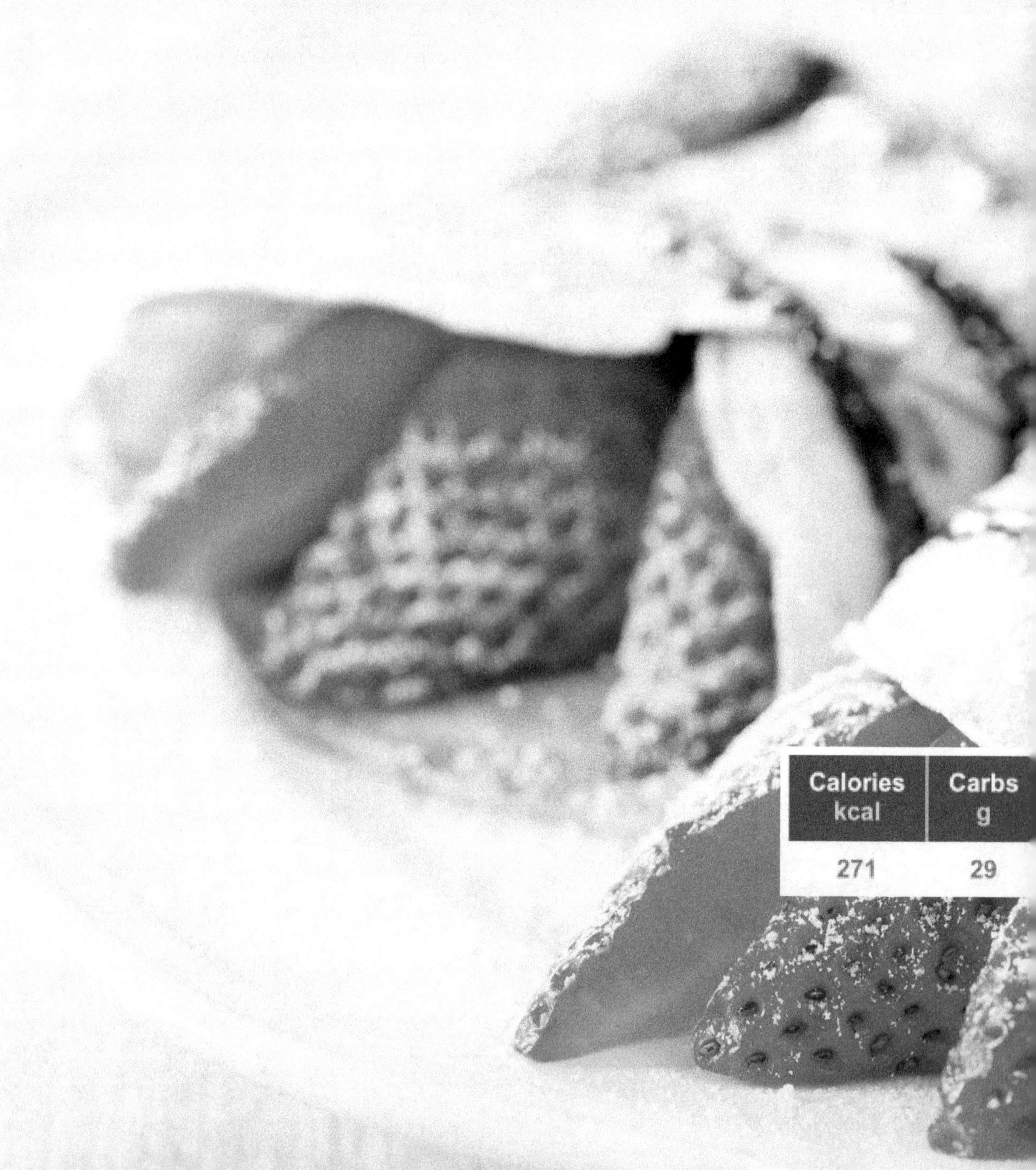

Calories kcal	Carbs g
271	29

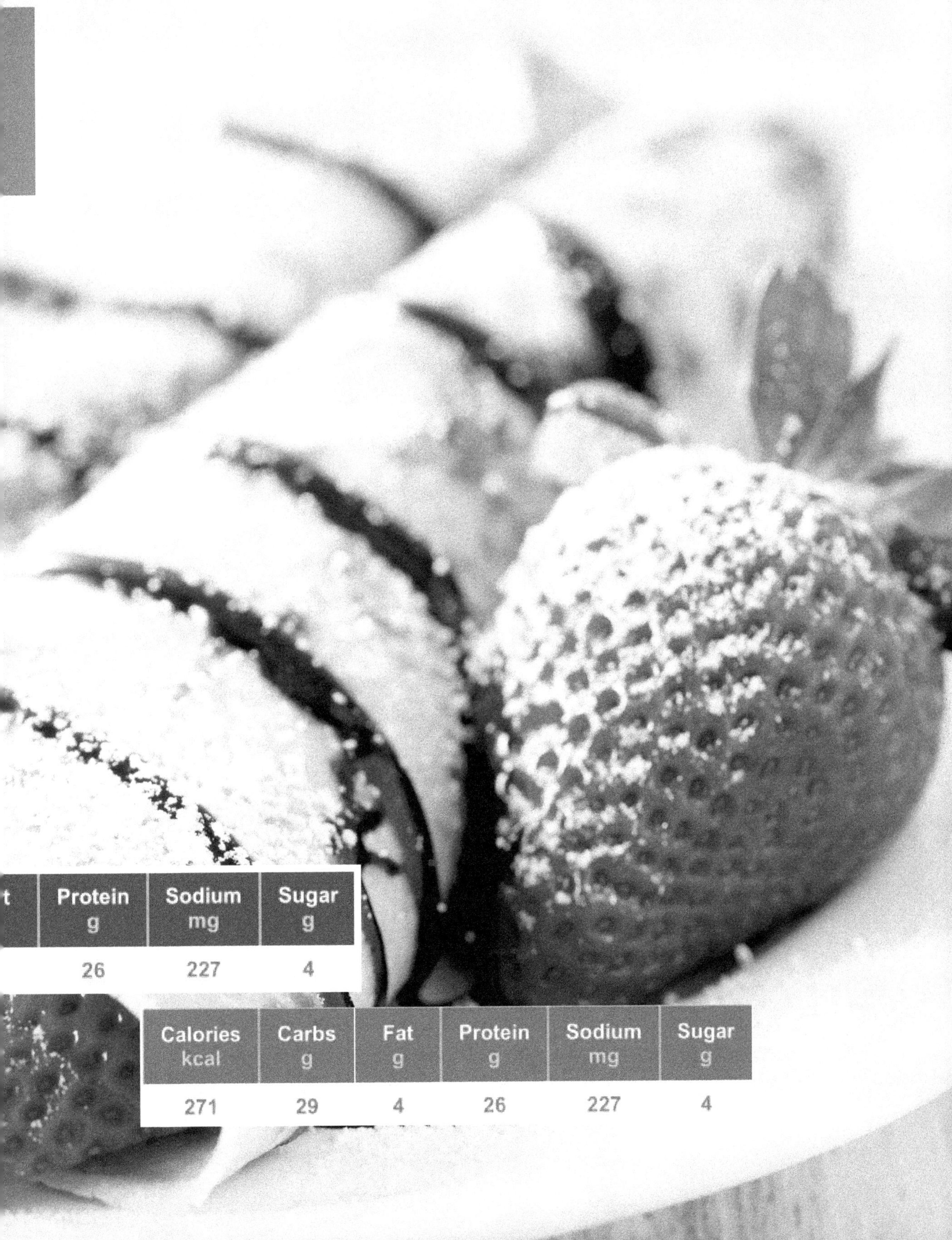

t	Protein g	Sodium mg	Sugar g
	26	227	4

Calories kcal	Carbs g	Fat g	Protein g	Sodium mg	Sugar g
271	29	4	26	227	4

STRAWBERRY CREPE

IDEAL POST WORKOUT SNACK 

INGREDIENTS

- 1/2 cup Fine Oats
- 30ml Unsweetened Almond Milk
- 15g Whey Protein Powder (low carb) Any flavour
- 3 egg whites
- 3 Whole Strawberries

Optional Extras: Stevia, Sugar free syrup, Honey, Himalayan sea salt, cinnamon

 POST WORKOUT MEAL

DIRECTIONS

Spray a pan with non-stck cooking spray and pre-heat on a low setting.

Blend together your oats, milk, protein powder and egg whites using an electric blender and add the batter to the pan.

Cook like a regular pancake, flipping once.

Slice up your strawberries and add to the middle of the pancake. Roll into a tasty wrap and finish with a splash of sugar-free syrup and stevia to taste.

BERRY BLAST SMOOTHIE

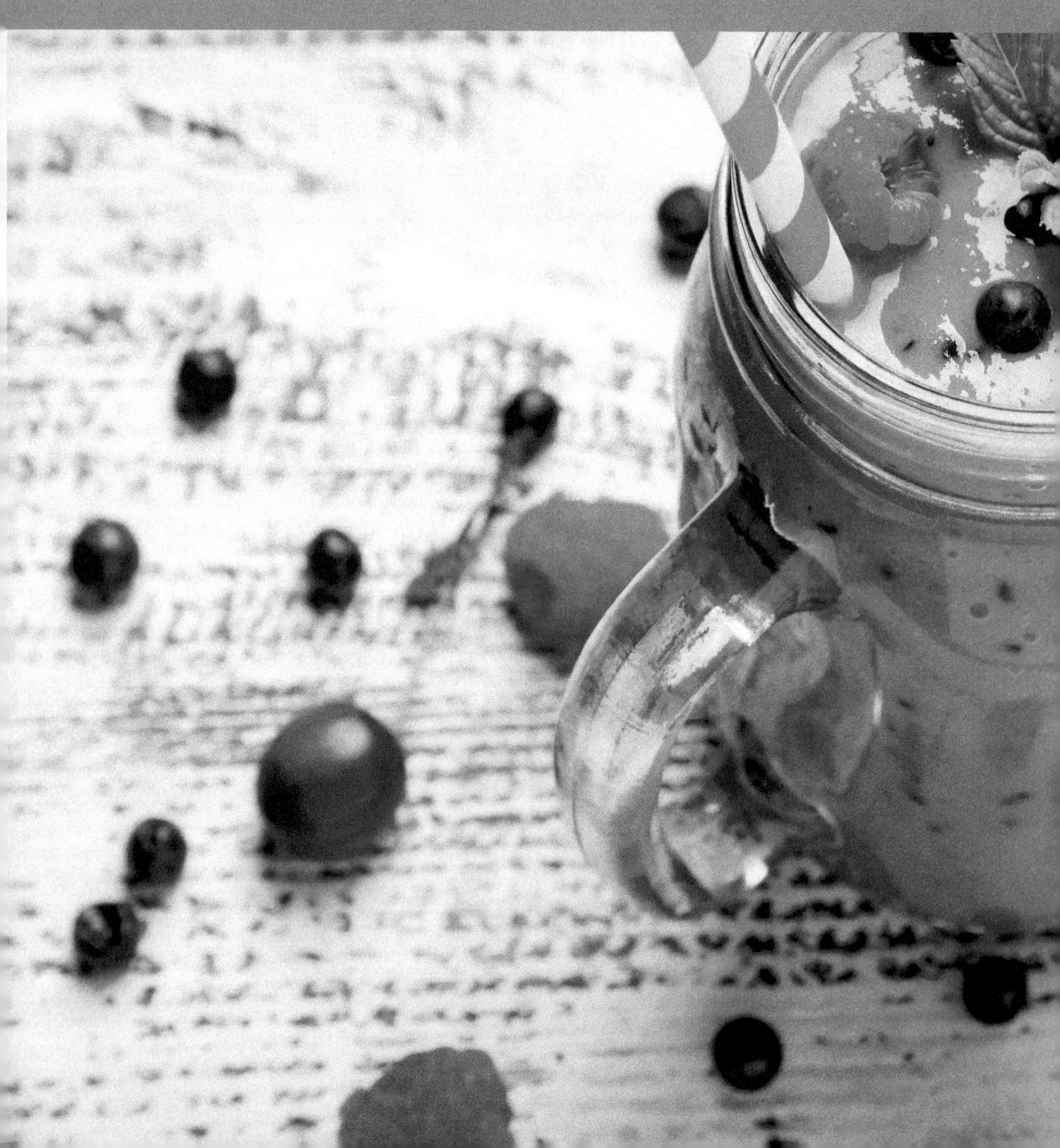

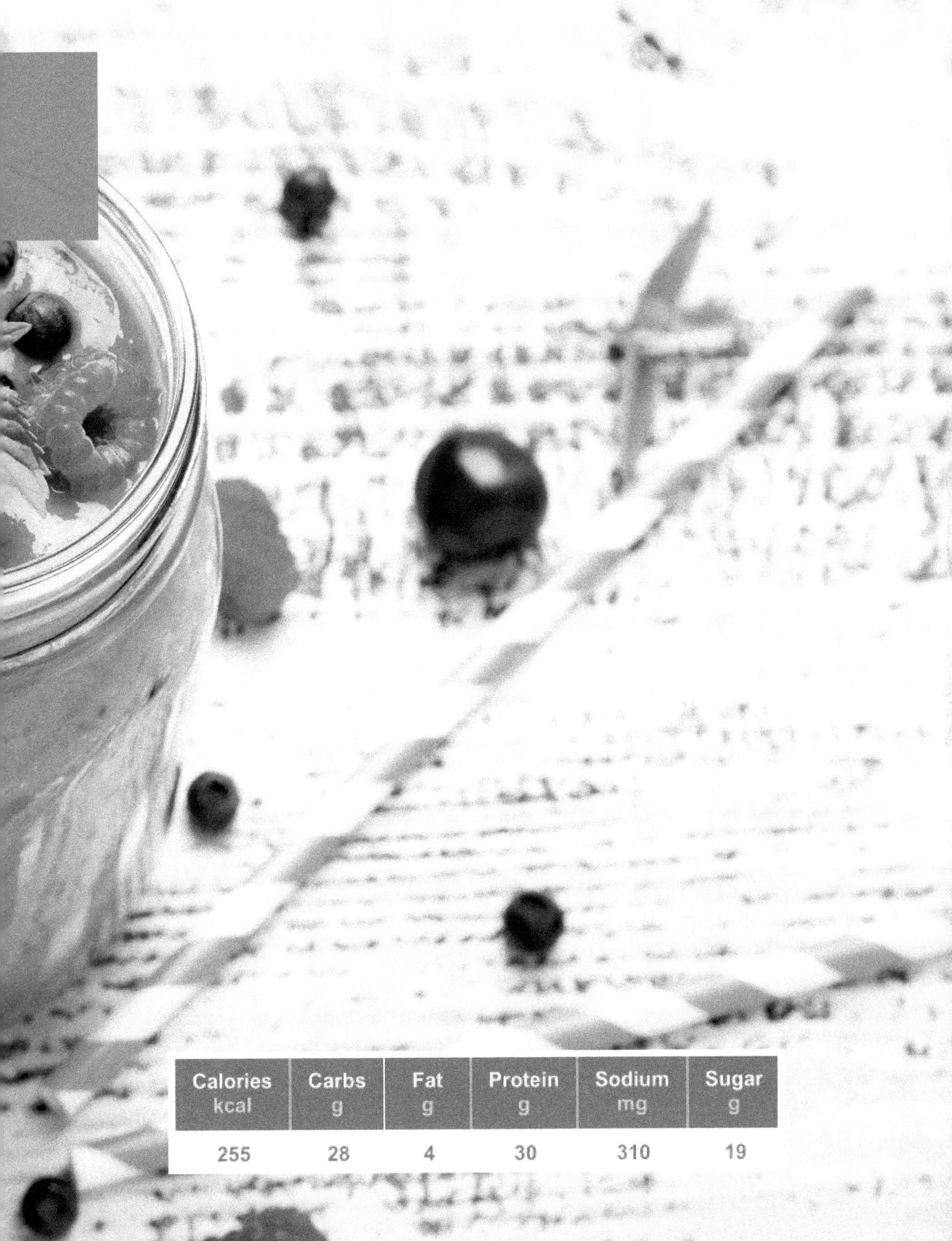

Calories kcal	Carbs g	Fat g	Protein g	Sodium mg	Sugar g
255	28	4	30	310	19

BERRY BLAST SMOOTHIE

IDEAL POST WORKOUT SNACK

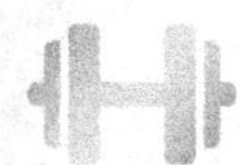

INGREDIENTS

» 1/2 cup Frozen Blueberries
» 3 Whole Strawberries
» 50g banana
» 200ml Unsweetened Almond Milk
» 30g Whey Protein Powder (low carb) Any flavour
» Ice cubes

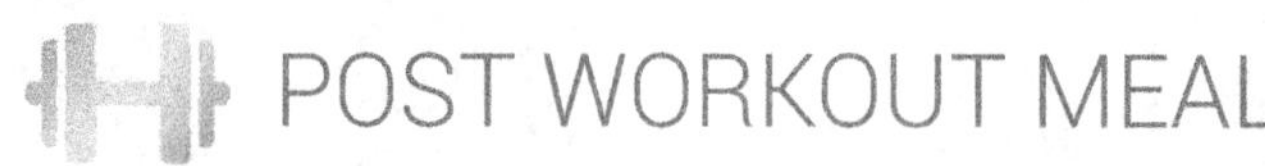

DIRECTIONS

Combine all ingredients into a food processor and pulse until the desired consistency is obtained.

Add more water if the consistency is too thick.

DIPPED BANANAS

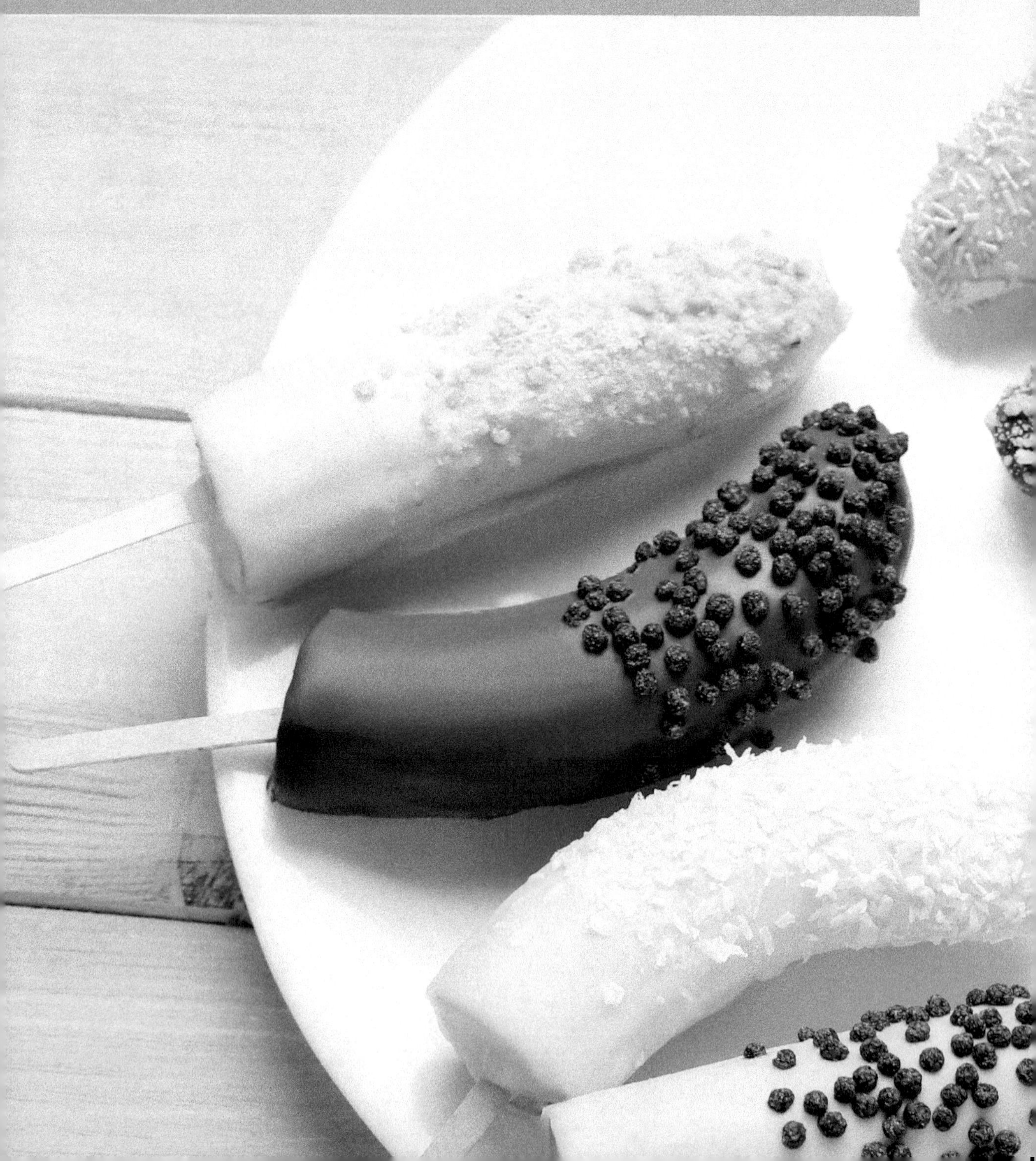

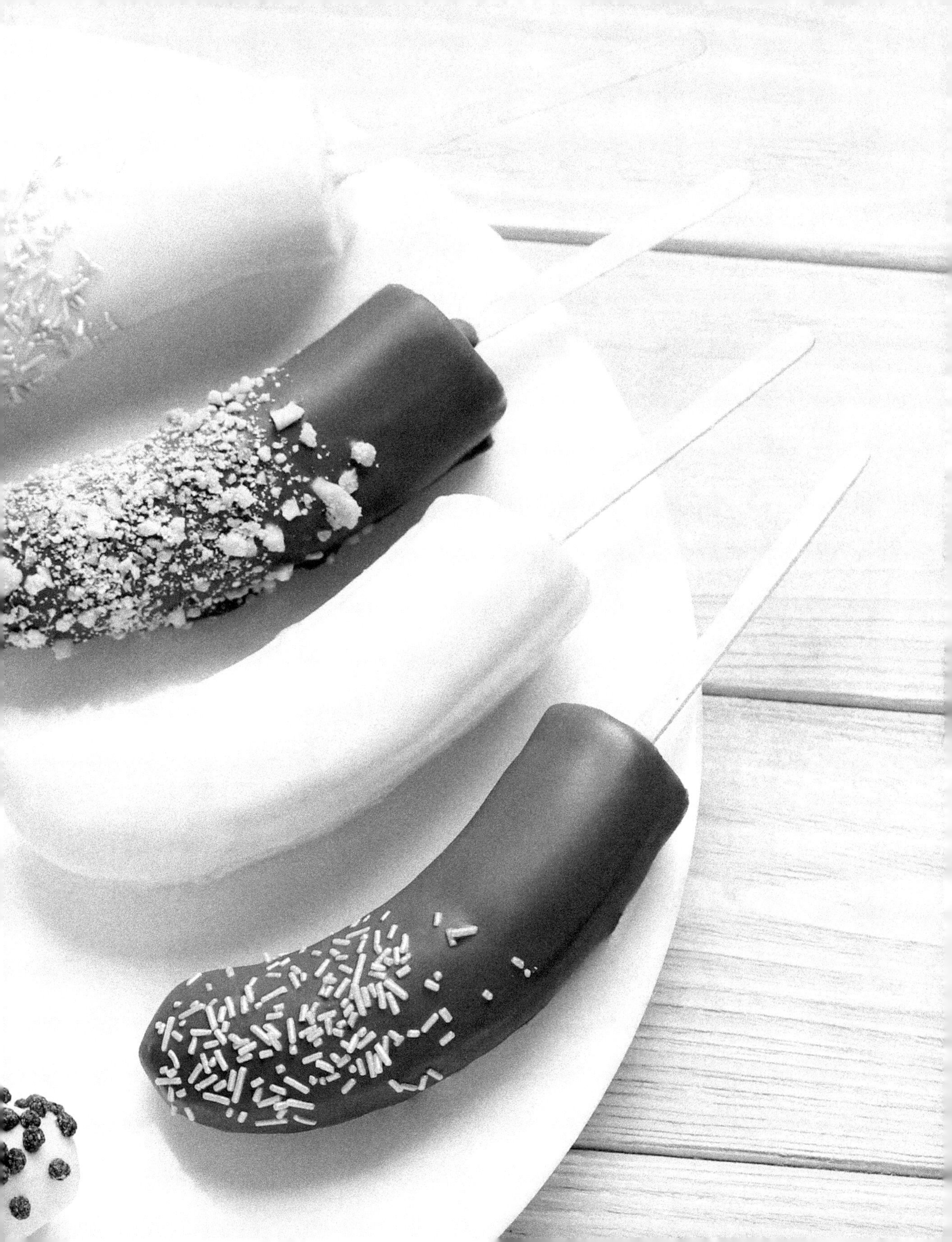

DIPPED STRAWBERRIES

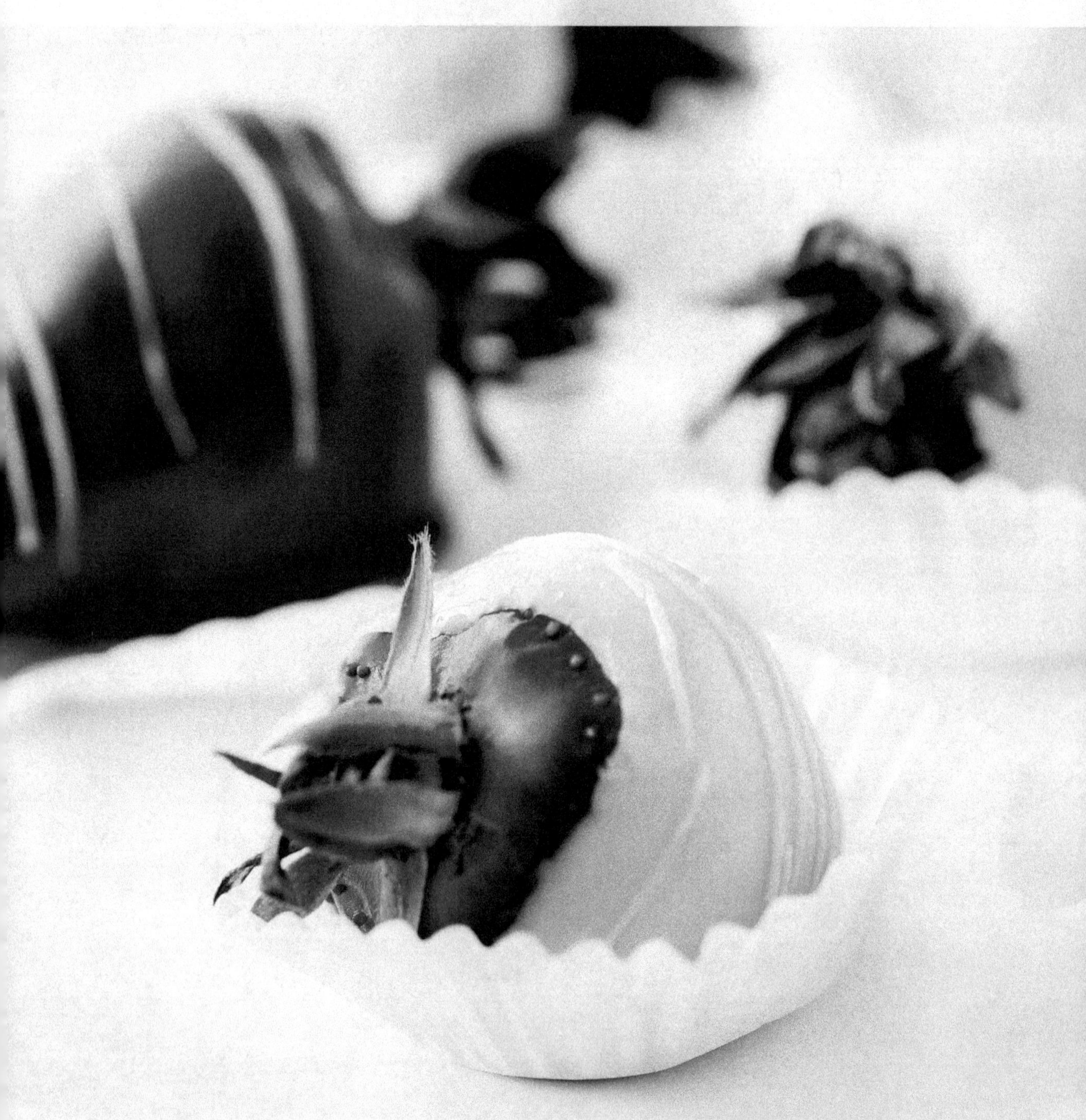

CPSIA information can be obtained
at www.ICGtesting.com
Printed in the USA
LVHW061712041019
633217LV00006B/147/P

9 781916 247178